W9-AAV-332

Structured Exercises in

WELLNESS

Promotion

Volume

3

Structured Exercises in

WELLNESS

Promotion

A Handbook for
Trainers, Educators, Group Leaders

Volume

3

**Edited by
Nancy Loving Tubesing, EdD
Donald A Tubesing, MDiv, PhD**

Copyright © 1986, 1994 by Whole Person Associates Inc.

REPRODUCTION POLICY

Unless otherwise noted, your purchase of this volume entitles you to reproduce a modest quantity of the worksheets that appear in this book for your education/training activities. For this limited worksheet reproduction no special additional permission is needed. However the following statement, in total, must appear on all copies that you reproduce.

> Reproduced from *Structured Exercises in Wellness Promotion, Volume 3*, Nancy Loving Tubesing and Donald A. Tubesing, Editors. © 1994 Whole Person Associates, 210 W Michigan, Duluth, MN 55802.

Specific prior written permission is required from the publisher for any reproduction of a complete or adapted exercise with trainer instructions, or large-scale reproduction of worksheets, or for inclusion of material in another publication. Licensing or royalty arrangement requests for this usage must be submitted in writing and approved prior to any such use.

For further information please write for our Permissions Guidelines and Standard Permissions Form. Permission requests must be submitted at least 30 days in advance of your scheduled printing or reproduction.

Library of Congress Cataloging in Publication Data

Structured exercises in wellness promotion : A handbook for trainers, educators, and
  group leaders / Nancy Loving Tubesing and Donald A. Tubesing, eds.
  192p. 23cm.
    Summary: A collection of thirty-six exercises for wellness promotion to be used
  by trainers and facilitators in group settings.
    ISBN 1-57025-020-0 (v.3 : pbk) : $29.95
    1. Health-Education, problems, exercises, etc. 2. Health—education and
  problems. I. Title. II. Tubesing, Nancy Loving III. Tubesing, Donald A.
  RA440.5.S77   1986, 1994
  613'.2—dc19   83-61074

Printed in the United States of America

10 9 8 7 6 5 4 3 2 1

Published by:

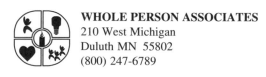

WHOLE PERSON ASSOCIATES
210 West Michigan
Duluth MN 55802
(800) 247-6789

PREFACE

Over a decade ago we launched an experiment in health education—the Whole Person series of **Structured Exercises in Wellness Promotion** and **Structured Exercises in Stress Management**. We believed that it was time to move beyond peptalks and handouts to an experiential approach that actively involves the participant—as a whole person—in the learning process.

What began as an experiment has become a catalyst for dramatic changes in health promotion and education! **Structured Exercises** volumes have found their way into the libraries of trainers, consultants, group workers, and health professionals around the world. We're proud that these volumes have become classics—the resource of choice for planning stress management and wellness promotion programs.

Our purpose in publishing this series was to foster inter-professional networking and to provide a framework though which we can all share our most effective ideas with each other. As you will soon discover, we scoured the country looking for the most innovative, effective teaching designs used by the most creative consultants and trainers in business, health care and social services, then included some of their most imaginative ideas in this volume.

Many of the exercises we designed ourselves and refined in hundreds of workshops we've conducted over the past twenty years. Some are new combinations of time-tested group process activities. Others were submitted by people like you who continually strive to add the creative touch to their teaching.

The layout of **Structured Exercises** is designed for easy photocopying of worksheets, handouts and preparation notes. Please take advantage of our generous policy for reproduction—but also please be fair to the creative individuals who have so generously shared their ideas with you.

☞ You may duplicate worksheets and handouts for use in training or educational events—as long as you use the proper citation as indicated on the copyright page. Please also give written credit to the original contributor. Whenever we've been able to track down the source of an idea, we've noted it. Please do the same when you share these ideas with others.

☞ However, all materials in this volume are still protected by copyright. Prior written permission from Whole Person Press is required if you plan large scale reproduction or distribution of *any portion of this book. If you wish to include any material or adaptation in another publication, you must have permission in writing before proceeding. Please send us your request and proposal at least thirty days in advance.*

Structured Exercises *are now available in two convenient formats. This small-format softcover version is produced with a new book binding process that stays open on your desk or podium for easy reference, and lies flat on the photocopier for quick duplication of worksheets.*

Many trainers enjoy the wide margins and larger type of the full-size looseleaf format, which provides plenty of space for you to add your own workshop designs, examples, chalktalk notes, and process reminders for your presentations. The looseleaf version also includes a complete package of camera-ready worksheet masters for easy reproduction of professional-looking handouts.

☞ *See page 156 in the Resources section for complete descriptions and ordering information for worksheet masters and companion volumes of the* **Stress** *and* **Wellness** *series in softcover and looseleaf formats.*

We are grateful to the many creative trainers who have so generously shared their "best" with you in this volume (see page 149) as well as others in the series. We hope that the ideas here stimulate your own creative juices.

So, go ahead. Strive to bring your teaching alive in new ways. Expand your stress management approach. Continue to touch and motivate people with learning experiences that engage and challenge them as whole persons.

Then let us know what works well for you. We'd love to consider your new ideas for inclusion in a future volume so that we can carry on the tradition of providing this international exchange of innovative teaching designs.

Duluth MN   *Nancy Loving Tubesing*
January 1994   *Donald A Tubesing*

INTRODUCTION

Wellness is the hot topic of the decade. If you're prepared to address the issue, you'll get plenty of opportunities. If you creatively involve people in the learning process, reflecting assessing, prioritizing, sorting, planning for change and affirming progress, your teaching will be much more helpful than even the most entertaining lecture.

Structured Exercises in Wellness Promotion, Volume 3 provides 36 designs you can use for getting people involved, whatever the setting and time constraints, whatever the sophistication of the audience. To aid you in the selection of appropriate content and process to meet your objectives, the exercises are grouped into five broad categories:

> ***Icebreakers:*** These short (10–20 minutes) exercises are designed to introduce people to each other and to open up participants' thinking process regarding wellness. They are lively! Each engages people actively in the topic and with each other. Try combining an icebreaker with an exercise from the wellness or self-care section for an instant evening progam.

> ***Wellness Exploration:*** These exercises explore the issue of wellness from the whole person perspective. Rather than focus merely on the physical, these processes help people examine their lifestyle. You'll find a mixture of moderate-length assessments (30–60 minutes) and major theme developers (60–90 minutes). Any exercise can easily be contracted or expanded to fit your purpose.

> ***Self-Care Strategies:*** These exercises promote personal responsibility for well-being. Participants examine their self-care patterns and explore specific self-care strategies in different life dimensions: physical (diet, relaxation, fitness), mental, rational, spiritual and lifestyle well-being. (10–60 minutes)

> ***Action Planning/Closure:*** These exercises help participants draw together their insights and determine the actions they wish to take on their own behalf. (20–40 minutes)

> ***Energizers:*** The energizers are designed to perk up the group whenever fatigue sets in. Sprinkle them throughout your program to illustrate skills or concepts. Try one for a change of pace—everyone's juices (including yours!) will be flowing again in 5–10 minutes.

The format is designed for easy use. You'll find that each exercise is described completely, including: goals, group size, time frame, materials needed, step-by-step process instructions, and variations.

   ☞ *Special instructions for the trainer and scripts to be read to the group are typed in italics.*

   ✔   Questions to ask the group are preceded by a check.

   ➤   Directions for group activities are indicated by an arrow.

   ●   Mini-lecture notes are preceded by a bullet.

Although the processes are primarily described for large group (25 to 100 people) workshop settings, most of the exercises work just as well with small groups, and many are appropriate for individual therapy or personal reflection.

If you are teaching in the workshop or large group setting, we believe that the use of small discussion groups is the most potent learning structure available to you. We've found that groups of four persons each provide ample air time and a good variety of interaction. If possible, let groups meet together two or three different times during the learning experience before forming new groups.

These personal sharing groups allow people to make positive contact with each other and encourage them to personalize their experience in depth. On evaluations, some people will say "Drop this," others will say, "Give us more small group time," but most will report that the time you give them to share with each other becomes the heart of the workshop.

If you are working with an intact group of 12 people or less, you may want to keep the whole group together for process and discussion time rather than divide into the suggested four or six person groups.

Each trainer has personal strengths, biases, pet concepts and processes. We expect and encourage you to expand and modify what you find here to accommodate your style. Adjust the exercises as you see fit. Bring these designs to life for your participants by inserting your own content and examples into your teaching. Experiment!

And when you come up with something new, let us know . . .

CONTENTS

WELLNESS EXPLORATION

SELF-CARE STRATEGIES

GROUP ENERGIZERS

RESOURCES

Icebreakers

73 INTRODUCTIONS 5

In these three quick ice-breakers participants introduce themselves as they exchange health tips (**My Mother Says**), share ways they sabotage well-being (**Sabotage and Self-Care**) and join in a follow-the-leader exercise/ stretch routine (**Simon Says**).

GOALS

To get acquainted.

To introduce subject matter that will be explored in more depth during the session.

TIME FRAME

10–15 minutes; with more than 20 participants, break up into small groups (4–12 persons) for introductions.

Introduction A: MY MOTHER SAYS

1) The trainer points out that each of us throughout our lifetime gathers a hodgepodge of aphorisms, admonitions, prohibitions and other folk wisdom about how to stay healthy and what we should do if we get sick (eg, "An apple a day keeps the doctor away," "Take two aspirin and go to bed," "Eat green vegetables," "Keep your feet dry," "Don't bother the doctor unless it's an emergency," etc).

   Participants are invited to recall some of the health-related messages they heard as children from parents, grandparents, relatives, neighbors, teachers, etc.

2) After a moment or two for "remembering," the trainer asks everyone to stand. The trainer then describes the process that participants should use as they move around the room and get acquainted with each other.

   ➤ Turn to a person near you, reach out and shake hands.

   ➤ As you clasp hands, introduce yourself and share a piece of advice from one of your childhood "experts on health."

   ➤ Use this format:

   ➤I'm   (your name)   and my   (mother/other source)   says . . .
          (words of wisdom/advice/caution)   !

©1994 Whole Person Press 210 W Michigan Duluth MN 55802   (800) 247-6789

➤ As soon as you have exchanged names and words of wisdom, move on and meet someone else. Try to recall a different health-related message each time you introduce yourself.

3) Participants are instructed to begin. After about 10 minutes the trainer stops the process and invites participants to share the most interesting advice they heard.

Introduction B: SABOTAGE AND SELF-CARE

1) The trainer asks participants to consider the variety of ways they undermine or sabotage their health (eg, smoking, suntanning, pigging out, disregarding pain, etc).

She then invites the group to think about all the health-enhancing ways they take care of themselves (eg, balanced meals, adequate rest, balancing work time and play time, exercise, intimate contact with loved ones, prayer, etc).

2) One by one participants introduce themselves, stating their name and sharing one sabotage style and one self-care technique they engage in that affects their well-being.

Introduction C: SIMON SAYS

1) The trainer announces that the group will get acquainted while exploring options for letting go of body tensions. He goes on to outline the three purposes of exercise: for flexibility, for strength and for aerobic (cardiovascular) conditioning.

The trainer challenges participants to think of several specific exercises of each type that the group could engage in together—given the space in the room and the attire of participants.

2) One-by-one participants take turns leading the group in different exercise/stretching activities using the **Simon Says** format (one minute each):

☞ *Challenge folks to stretch different muscle groups so that the whole body gets a workout.*

➤ The "leader" comes to the front and introduces himself:
  ➤ "I am _____ (leader's name) _____."

©1994 Whole Person Press 210 W Michigan Duluth MN 55802   (800) 247-6789

> ➤ The leader describes and demonstrates his exercise.
> ➤ The leader invites the group to join, saying, " (leader's name) says do this with me!"
> ➤ After about a minute, the leader chooses someone else to be leader.

> ☞ *The trainer should lead the first one-minute segment; the process continues with a succession of leaders until all have been introduced and have led their exercise.*

VARIATION

■ With more than 20 people, break into smaller groups and assign a different body part (eg, neck, back, feet, etc) to each team. Participants each devise an exercise for that area, introduce themselves and teach their exercise to the others in the team. Each team chooses their favorite from those presented and when the trainer indicates, they introduce it to the large group using the **Simon Says** format.

TRAINER'S NOTES

74 SATURDAY NIGHT LIVE!

In this dramatic ice-breaker, small groups of participants dream up amusing skits in which they introduce themselves to the whole group.

GOALS

To promote interaction and help people get acquainted.

GROUP SIZE

Unlimited; described for 30 participants.

TIME FRAME

20–30 minutes; longer with larger groups.

PROCESS

1) The trainer asks participants to "number off" (1-2-3-4-5-6, etc) and designates a spot in the room for each group to gather.

    ☞ *This process works best with about 6 people per group. Adjust your number of groups accordingly.*

2) After everyone is settled, she announces that groups will have about 15 minutes to get acquainted with each other and to prepare a 3-minute skit that will introduce all the members of their group to the other participants.

    ☞ *If you are worried about putting people under too much pressure, you may want to suggest a theme for the skits, such as TV formats (eg, game show, talk show, interviews, etc). But most audiences have more than enough creativity to generate their own!*

3) After 10–15 minutes, the trainer reconvenes the participants around the "stage" area and announces the order for skit presentations (eg, 5's first, then 4's, 3's, 2's and 1's).

    One-by-one, the groups introduce themselves "on stage!"

Submitted by Sandy Queen.

TRAINER'S NOTES

75 HEALTH-ORIENTED PEOPLE HUNT

In this lively get-acquainted contest participants gather signatures from their wellness-oriented neighbors.

GOALS

To facilitate intermingling among participants.

To promote sharing of personal health-oriented information by participants.

GROUP SIZE

Any group size is appropriate, as long as there is adequate space for participants to circulate freely.

TIME FRAME

15–20 minutes

MATERIALS NEEDED

A copy of the **Health-Oriented People Hunt Contest** worksheet for each participant.

PROCESS

1) The trainer introduces the contest rules and procedures to be followed by participants.

➤ You are about to engage in a contest to discover the self-care secrets and health-oriented behaviors represented in this group.

➤ Each person will receive a list of 20 items that may be true of one or more participants.

➤ You will have about 10 minutes to find people for whom these items are true. Try to find someone for each item. When you find an appropriate person, get his or her signature, and ask the related bonus question (see worksheet). Record any pertinent information below the signature.

➤ You may sign your name to one item that is true for you. Don't forget to answer the bonus question!

➤ People and items may be matched in any order—but you must find a different person for each item.

➤ The first person to complete all items will win the contest, if—and only if—the winner can also introduce and identify each person who signed his or her sheet.

2) The trainer supplies each participant with a **Health-Oriented People Hunt Contest** worksheet and then signals them to circulate and obtain as many different signatures as possible. (10 minutes)

The participant with the first completed worksheet or the one with the most names when time is called is the contest winner.

3) The trainer announces the "winner" and asks her to introduce the health-oriented people she found.

☞ *If the "winner" gets stuck on any item, ask for a volunteer who can introduce a health-oriented person who fulfills the item requirements.*

After everyone is introduced, a "brown bag" surprise (sufficient quantity of sugar-free gum or candy to share with everyone) is awarded to the winner.

VARIATIONS

■ With more than 30 people, divide participants into 2 groups and conduct simultaneous contests.

■ In a small group, participants may use one person for more than one question, but they should try to interact with each person at least once.

■ Participants can be asked to generate additional contest items for group discussion or for inclusion in future worksheets.

Submitted by Kent Beeler

©1994 Whole Person Press 210 W Michigan Duluth MN 55802   (800) 247-6789

HEALTH-ORIENTED PEOPLE HUNT CONTEST

Circulate around the group introducing yourself and looking for people who fit these descriptions. Discuss the appropriate contest items and answer the related bonus questions, then exchange signatures.

FIND SOMEONE WHO . . .   **SIGNATURE**

1) Follows a balanced diet and eats meals regularly.   _____

   Bonus: Where did you learn this habit and how long has it been a part of your lifestyle?

2) Quit smoking within the past year and remained a non-smoker for at least three months   _____

   Bonus: Where do you still feel the urge for a smoke and how do you deal with it?

3) Reduced consumption of caffeine or alcohol within the past year.   _____

   Bonus: What influenced you to cut down?

4) Lost (and kept off) at least 10 pounds within the past year.   _____

   Bonus: How did you accomplish this feat?

5) Gets adequate amount of restful sleep at least six nights a week.   _____

   Bonus: What happens when you don't get enough rest?

6) Uses relaxation techniques (biofeedback, meditation, quiet reflection, etc.) at least 3 times a week.   _____

   Bonus: What technique(s) do you find most effective?

7) Regularly makes out a "to do" list and completes nearly all the day's activities listed.   _____

   Bonus: How do you deal with interruptions and emergencies?

8) Exercises actively (jogging, aerobics, cycling, walking) for 20-30 minutes at least 3 times a week.   _____

   Bonus: What advice would you give people who are just starting out on an exercise program?

9) Has a healthy self-concept.   _____

    Bonus: *How do you handle mistakes or criticism?*

10) Uses seat belts whenever possible.   _____

    Bonus: *What convinced you to use seat belts?*

11) Operates vehicles only when not under the influence of alcohol or other drugs.   _____

    Bonus: *How do you manage situations where the driver (you or someone else) has indulged in alcohol or drugs?*

12) Finds it easy to laugh at self.   _____

    Bonus: *What helps you to keep life in perspective?*

13) Manages the stress in his/her life well.   _____

    Bonus: *What coping strategies are the most successful for you?*

14) Has experienced a dramatic life-changing event. _____

    Bonus: *What did you learn from the experience and how has it affected your well-being?*

15) Regularly finds an outlet for his/her creativity. _____

    Bonus: *What is the outlet and what special benefits do you receive from this creative expression?*

16) Has intentionally chosen a physician who has a wellness philosophy.   _____

    Bonus: *How did you find this person?*

17) Is in a support group of some kind.   _____

    Bonus: *What needs does this group fulfill for you?*

18) Maintains a healthy balance between investments in work, home and self.   _____

    Bonus: *What would you say is the key to finding a healthy balance?*

19) Has a sense of spiritual depth, commitment and guidance in their life.   _____

    Bonus: *How does this spiritual force affect your total well-being?*

©1994 Whole Person Press 210 W Michigan Duluth MN 55802   (800) 247-6789

76 PART OF ME

Participants use meaningful items brought from home to introduce themselves and to reflect on the underlying values that influence their self-care choices.

GOALS

To promote self-disclosure and interaction among participants.

To identify and share personal values with other group members.

To raise consciousness about the role of values in shaping health-related attitudes and behaviors.

GROUP SIZE

Unlimited.

TIME FRAME

2–3 minutes per person

PROCESS

☞ *This exercise requires some advance preparation. Ask participants to bring something (a song, poem, object, etc) of special significance to share with others at this meeting.*

1) The trainer announces that it is time to unveil the meaningful items participants have brought to the meeting. He asks everyone to take out their "special something" and prepare to share it with the group by describing its significance.

   ☞ *If anyone has forgotten to bring an item, she can tell about a significant quotation, song, story or poem—or choose to describe something she is wearing that has special meaning.*

2) One at a time participants share with the group why they chose the item they did and how it reflects their underlying values.

3) After all participants have completed their opportunity for "show and tell," the trainer explains the importance to well-being of reflecting on personal values. He notes that values are the core criteria that influence decision-making in all areas of life—including health.

©1994 Whole Person Press 210 W Michigan Duluth MN 55802   (800) 247-6789

The trainer invites participants to recall and list the values represented by the collection of objects the group brought to share. As each value is suggested, the trainer records it on the board and asks the group to describe how that particular value might play a role in shaping our self-care attitudes and behaviors.

4) In conclusion, the trainer asks the group to brainstorm an additional list of other values that might influence health-related behaviors and uses this information as a bridge to the next content segment.

VARIATIONS

■ Instead of focusing on values, the choice of items for "show and tell" can be geared to fit other possible objectives. With an intact staff, ask people to bring an item that symbolizes a specific need to which they would like others in the group to respond. Or participants could bring something that represents an area in their life they are currently working to improve.

■ This exercise can serve as an introduction to other team-building experiences geared toward improving staff relationships.

TRAINER'S NOTES

Submitted by Mark Warner.

©1994 Whole Person Press 210 W Michigan Duluth MN 55802   (800) 247-6789

77 GETTING TO KNOW YOU

Participants share their philosophy of health and affirm personal wellness goals, as they introduce themselves to several others in the group.

GOALS

To articulate a personal philosophy of wellness.

To establish goals for personal well-being.

To stimulate group cohesion.

GROUP SIZE

Unlimited, as long as there is space for participants to move around the room and pair up with one another.

TIME FRAME

20–30 minutes

MATERIALS NEEDED

One 3x5 index card for each participant.

PROCESS

1) The trainer distributes 3x5 index cards to participants and gives instructions.

   ☞ *Don't rush! Explain the items as necessary and give examples. Pause long enough between each item so people have ample time for reflection and writing.*

   ➤ Write your name on the card.

   ➤ Compose a brief self-introduction—write a few sentences about yourself.

   ➤ Briefly summarize your definition of health/wellness.

   ➤ List your personal wellness goals.

2) Participants are directed to seek out someone whom they either do not know or wish to know better, and to spend about 5 minutes with this person sharing the information on their cards.

©1994 Whole Person Press 210 W Michigan Duluth MN 55802   (800) 247-6789

3) After 3–5 minutes, the trainer calls time and directs participants to find new partners and repeat *Step 2*. This process is repeated several times, each time with a new partner.

4) The trainer collects everyone's cards and utilizes the information they provide about participants in planning the remainder of the session/ workshop to meet the individual needs and goals of participants.

TRAINER'S NOTES

Submitted by Marcia A Schnorr.

©1994 Whole Person Press 210 W Michigan Duluth MN 55802   (800) 247-6789

78 GALLOPING GOURMET

Participants introduce themselves as a favorite meal and then join in trios to calculate and compare calorie content.

GOALS

To get acquainted.

To identify food preferences and expose their calorie content.

GROUP SIZE

Unlimited.

TIME FRAME

20–30 minutes

MATERIALS NEEDED

3x5 cards for all; for every 3 participants a chart or book outlining the calorie content of common foods, including popular fast foods.

PROCESS

1) The trainer distributes a blank 3x5 note card to each person and asks participants to write down on one side their *favorite fruit, favorite vegetable,* and *favorite candy bar.*

   After a moment for writing, the trainer invites people to identify their favorite meal and to write it down on the other side of the card, describing this special treat in as much detail as possible.

   ☞ *Encourage people to remember favorite foods from childhood, comfort foods, celebration foods, home-cooked foods, restaurant specialties. Ask, "What does your mother fix on special occasions such as holidays or birthdays? What do you crave when you're under stress?"*

2) After 2 or 3 minutes for recalling and recording culinary favorites, participants are directed to stand up and mill around the room until they find two other people who chose the same fruit, vegetable or candy bar that they did.

©1994 Whole Person Press 210 W Michigan Duluth MN 55802   (800) 247-6789

☞ *Pairs or quartets could be substituted for trios.*

The trainer announces that as soon as participants find two other compatriots, the trio should pull chairs together, sit down and introduce themselves describing their favorite meal to each other in vivid detail (2–3 minutes).

3) As the trios are winding up their introductions, the trainer interrupts the discussion and asks everyone to write down an estimate of the calorie content of their favorite meal and the favorite foods chosen by the others in their trio.

The trainer distributes a calorie chart/book to each group. She instructs trios to use this resource to determine the total calories included in their favorite meal. Each person records his total on his note card.

☞ *Encourage participants to work together so that they maximize opportunities to learn various calorie counts. Be prepared to help clarify portion sizes and, if necessary, estimate calorie content of foods not included in the charts.*

4) After about 5 minutes, the trainer reconvenes the whole group and determines the calorie range represented, asking questions such as:

✔ How many people's special delight was over 1,000 calories? Over 1,500? Over 2,000?

✔ How many people's favorite meal was under 1,000 calories? Under 500? Under 100?

She also inquires about how accurately participants estimated the calorie content of their own and other's favorite foods:

✔ How many people **over**estimated the calorie content of your own meal or snack? How many **under**estimated?

✔ How many people **over**estimated the calorie content of another person's meal? How many **under**estimated a colleague's calorie content?

5) The trainer comments on the group's patterns of food preference and knowledge of calorie counts. Participants are also invited to share observations.

©1994 Whole Person Press 210 W Michigan Duluth MN 55802   (800) 247-6789

TRAINER'S NOTES

©1994 Whole Person Press 210 W Michigan Duluth MN 55802   (800) 247-6789

Wellness
Exploration

79 PERSONAL WELLNESS WHEEL

Participants inventory themselves on eight dimensions of wellness, affirming the areas of strength and noting those areas needing additional attention.

GOALS

To assess participants' current level of wellness on eight dimensions: intellectual, emotional, physical, social, vocational, environmental, psychological and spiritual.

To share ideas for maintaining personal well-being in areas of strength and improving those areas where deficiencies are evident.

GROUP SIZE

Unlimited. Also works well with individuals.

TIME FRAME

15–20 minutes

MATERIALS NEEDED

Blackboard or newsprint easel; copy of the **Personal Wellness Wheel** worksheet for each participant.

PROCESS

1) The trainer opens this exercise by mentioning that wellness is a multi-dimensional concept involving the whole person.

   On a blackboard or newsprint, he lists eight aspects of wellness: intellectual, emotional, physical, social, vocational, environmental, psychological and spiritual. The trainer enlists the group's help in building a working list of the attributes that define each dimension of well-being. (5 minutes)

2) The trainer makes an analogy between wellness (a wheel) and its various dimensions (spokes) that support it and keep it balanced.
   - A bicycle would not work well if it were to try to roll on the hub of the wheel. The small hub would ride too roughly. It would get stuck in the first small hole it encountered and would gouge itself to a stop! Therefore, the rim and tire is suspended by spokes far out from the hub.

©1994 Whole Person Press 210 W Michigan Duluth MN 55802   (800) 247-6789

These many spokes of the same size and length are carefully balanced; each contributes its share to supporting the larger rim and tire which easily can roll over the bumps in the road. If too many spokes on one side are damaged, the wheel will collapse, and the bicycle will no longer work.

● So also with wellness. **Each dimension (spoke) needs our attention.** If all the various qualities of wellness are poorly developed, we end up with a very small wheel—one that rolls poorly and quickly gets stuck in the small ruts it encounters. If some of the qualities of wellness (spokes) are developed more than others, we're in for a lopsided "galumpity" ride!

● **We need to develop all aspects** (spokes) of our well-being in order to roll safely and effectively over the obstacles and pitfalls of life. A balance of well-being in all dimensions of life is our best insurance for maintaining long term vitality.

3) Each participant receives a copy of the **Personal Wellness Wheel** worksheet and the trainer gives instructions for completing it.

➤ On the worksheet the eight dimensions of wellness are depicted as different spokes on a wheel. Each spoke contains a continuum for measuring well-being in that dimension.

☞ *Ask the group to brainstorm health factors in each of the eight dimensions, or give several examples yourself:*

+ ***spiritual*** *(faith, values, meditation, worship, etc);*
+ ***environmental*** *(resources, conservation, pollution, etc);*
+ ***emotional*** *(feelings, self-esteem, moods, etc);*
+ ***psychological*** *(stress, coping, problem-solving, etc);*
+ ***social*** *(relationships, family, community, etc).*

Participants can jot down the relevant factors for each dimension on their own worksheets.

➤ Consider each continuum and place a dot on the line at the point that represents your current "health" position on that factor.

Dots placed closest to the hub indicate areas for attention and growth. Dots placed further from the hub, toward the outer edge, indicate areas of well-being (The Ideal).

☞ *Give people time to finish this step before proceeding to the next.*

©1994 Whole Person Press 210 W Michigan Duluth MN 55802   (800) 247-6789

➤ Connect the dots and examine the "pattern" of well-being that emerges for you.

➤ Then complete the summary observation questions on the second worksheet.

4) The trainer invites participants to share reactions and comments about the configuration of their personal wellness wheels. If the following points do not emerge from the ensuing discussion, the trainer may want to be sure they are covered.

● Wellness is a complicated and multi-faceted concept involving far more than just physical health.

● None of us is perfect. We all have areas of strength and areas that could use improvement.

● Dimensions of life in which we are particularly healthy can often help us compensate for those dimensions in which we are hurting.

● Optimal well-being challenges us to move as much as possible toward a balance of healthfulness in every aspect of our lives. Only then will we be able to roll with whatever crosses our path.

VARIATIONS

■ The **Personal Wellness Wheel** could be cut out and glued to heavy stock cardboard. A board game is made by inserting an arrow spinner in the hub. Participants take turns spinning the arrow. As they land on a spoke, participants briefly describe their status on that wellness dimension and what they might do to enhance it.

■ As part of *Step 4*, participants who have registered near the ideal on one or more dimensions of the **Personal Wellness Wheel** can congregate with those whose assessment is less positive. The interchange can focus on ways participants can reach or maintain a more positive health status on different dimensions.

■ For smaller groups, the trainer can enlarge the **Personal Wellness Wheel** and plot a group composite profile, taking care to preserve anonymity. Each individual can then compare his own profile to the group norm.

*This exercise, suggested to us by Kent Beeler, is adapted from **The Wellness Series I booklet** (1983) produced by Mennonite Mutual Aid, 1110 North Main Street PO Box 483 Goshen IN 46526. For copies of this booklet or others in their excellent wellness series, please contact them directly.*

PERSONAL WELLNESS WHEEL

a dot-to-dot activity

Directions:

1. Place a dot on each spoke (line) on the **Personal Wellness Wheel** indicating where you feel you are now.
2. Connect the dots.
3. The distance between your spoke and the rim—the wellness "ideal"— indicates opportunities for personal growth and development.

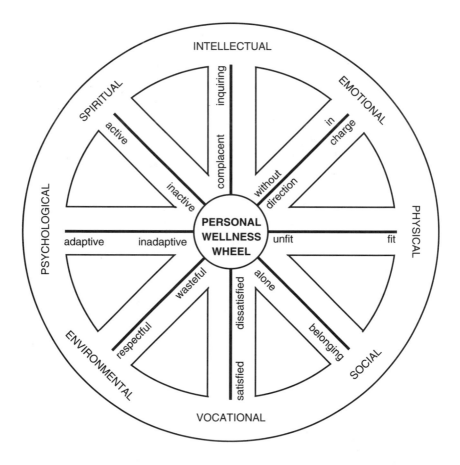

This activity has been adapted from **Wellness Series 1** (Goshen IN: Mennonite Mutual Aid, 1983).

©1994 Whole Person Press 210 W Michigan Duluth MN 55802   (800) 247-6789

PERSONAL WELLNESS WHEEL: OBSERVATIONS

In which dimensions of life are you most well?

In which are you least well?

Comment on the pattern you see in your well-being profile.
Is your Wheel round? Lopsided? Would your Wheel *roll*?

How do you feel about what you see?

How well do the patterns you see correspond to what you expected to see?

What improvements, if any, would you like to see in your Wheel profile?

List two or three immediate steps you could take to round out your Wheel and make these improvements.

©1994 Whole Person Press 210 W Michigan Duluth MN 55802   (800) 247-6789

80 WELLNESS CULTURE TEST

Participants examine the influence of their environment on their personal wellness habits by answering Ardell's tongue-in-cheek wellness culture test and discussing the serious issues that it raises. They then take steps to reshape their cultural norms in a health-enhancing direction.

GOALS

To illustrate the force that cultural norms exert over our lifestyle decisions.

To analyze assumptions about the proper and healthful way to live.

To facilitate the development of positive health-enhancing norms.

GROUP SIZE

Unlimited.

TIME REQUIRED

60–90 minutes

MATERIALS NEEDED

One copy of the **Ardell Wellness Culture Test** for each participant. A blackboard or newsprint easel for each small group of 6 to 8 people (or newsprint can be hung on the wall around the room).

PROCESS

1) The trainer introduces the idea that our culture is a powerful shaper of behavior.

- Where do we learn to live? to behave? to celebrate? to work? to play? etc. We watch! We watch our parents, our friends and our heroes. We watch television, read the newspaper and listen to the radio . . . and we learn how to fit in! We learn what is normal!

- Unfortunately, many of the ways we are taught by these sources to behave are almost guaranteed to make us sick. To celebrate, we learn to eat sweets and drink alcohol. We learn to grind it out at work in order to be successful. We learn to ignore our feelings. We learn to get by on less sleep. We learn to smoke and to drink coffee. We learn these and thousands of other habits simply by watching those around us and imitating their behavior.

©1994 Whole Person Press 210 W Michigan Duluth MN 55802   (800) 247-6789

- It is clear that the major current American health epidemics are not the result of fate, an ill wind, or a bug. They are primarily related to the way we live. We seldom catch our death of anything anymore. We get it the old fashioned way—*We earn it!*
- There is a big difference between "average American," "normal human," and "possible American/human." The ways we have learned to live are not the only options. We can challenge what we have been taught. We can rethink our patterns of living and set some new norms for ourselves and perhaps even our neighbors.

2) The trainer distributes a copy of the **Ardell Wellness Culture Test** to each participant and instructs them to complete the quiz answering "yes" or "no" to each statement of "What's normal around here?"

   ☞ *Decide in advance if you want participants to focus on a particular environment such as home, recreation group, the work place or even their department. If not, suggest that they respond according to the composite of environments, in general, within which they live.*

3) As soon as most people have completed the quiz, the trainer invites participants to make up their own scoring system, determining what total of "yes" answers is good, poor, horrible, etc. Once they have devised a scoring system for themselves, participants use it to interpret their own results and write themselves recommendations (like a teacher's notes in a term paper).

   ☞ *Ardell's scoring system goes like this:*
   > *5 "yes" = Big trouble*
   > *8 "yes" = Undertaker city*
   > *10 "yes" = Everlasting hangnail and tooth decay*
   > *Encourage your participants to be as creative.*

4) The trainer divides participants into groups of 6–8 people, and instructs them to briefly describe the scoring systems they created and to report on the results they achieved based on this scoring standard. (2 minutes each—15 minutes total)

5) Groups are instructed to come to a consensus, listing in rank order the five items in the **Ardell Wellness Culture Test** that are the most destructive within the cultural environments represented by the group members. (10 minutes)

©1994 Whole Person Press 210 W Michigan Duluth MN 55802   (800) 247-6789

The trainer announces the rules for this consensus-building:

➤ Everyone must have a chance to be heard.

➤ No voting or "averaging" is allowed. Group consensus must be reached based on debate only.

➤ All must agree with the selection and the ranking.

☞ *The purpose of this exercise is to stimulate among participants an energetic give and take about the cultural factors. If the rules are scrupulously followed, consensus will never be reached. By the end of the ten minutes, however, each group should select and rank their five items.*

You may want to give them a two minute warning before closure, so that they select a list of five items to work with in the next step.

6) Groups are invited to experiment with changing the five destructive cultural norms they have selected. The trainer gives instructions for the group discussion.

➤ List on newsprint or blackboard the five "culprit" norms you have selected.

➤ Then consider each norm and discuss the following questions. (10 minutes total)

➤ What would it be like if this norm were not "normal" around here?

➤ What would people do for fun? for success? for transportation? for contact? How would they deal with their feelings? spend their day? etc.

☞ *You may want to display these questions on newsprint for easy reference.*

7) After about 10 minutes the trainer challenges the groups to counteract each of their 5 norms that promote "sick-being" with one or more alternative norms that would promote well-being. These new, more positive norms are listed on newsprint. (5 minutes)

☞ *Encourage participants to be as specific as possible in developing new norms. For example, to replace the norm that requires sweets and alcohol for celebration, the group might suggest a group back rub, followed by a cheer, followed by a snake dance around the block with a friendly wave to all passers-by!*

8) The trainer asks the groups to choose their most creative wellness-promoting norm and prepare to describe/demonstrate it to the whole class.

> ➤ Devise a strategy for involving the entire class in practicing the new norm you are recommending.

> ➤ Select one person to present your group's idea.

9) The trainer reconvenes the entire group and invites a representative of each small group to describe a few of the new health-promoting norms they have developed. Each representative leads the total group in actively participating—right then and there—in one of the new norms they are recommending!

> ☞ *Everyone should get involved in trying the health-enhancing activities that up until this point have "not been normal around here."*

10) The trainer asks for comments on insights and observations that have occurred to participants during this norm-breaking exercise.

VARIATION

> ■ *Pathology of Normalcy* (**Wellness 3**, p 29) would be an effective warmup or closing to this process.

*Submitted by Donald B Ardell. This test was originally inspired by the writings of Robert F Allen, PhD whose landmark book **Lifegain** provided the foundation for all subsequent work in identifying and changing hazardous cultural norms.*

ARDELL WELLNESS CULTURE TEST

Answer "yes" or "no" to the following statements—each of which begins with the phrase, "It's normal around here to . . ."

It's normal around here . . .	*Yes*	*No*
1) To celebrate special occasions with sweets or alcohol or both.	❏	❏
2) To drink coffee throughout the day because it's so readily available.	❏	❏
3) To not wear seat belts, to not exercise daily and to eat junk food.	❏	❏
4) To ignore the 55 mph speed limit, stop signs and traffic lights if it looks like you can get away with it.	❏	❏
5) To tolerate tobacco odors and smoke because smokers have rights too, and you don't want to be pushy or a crank.	❏	❏
6) To think you're weird if you take time out to close your eyes and relax several times throughout the day to balance or calm yourself.	❏	❏
7) To take pills or go to a doctor when you are not feeling well, or to pass out aspirins and other medications to each other.	❏	❏
8) To avoid expressing feelings because that makes you seem strange.	❏	❏
9) To get positive reinforcement for being rushed, harried, or drawn in appearance because the more harried you appear, the harder you must be working.	❏	❏
10) To complain a lot—about the job, the boss, the weather, the President, the economy, each other, the food, local teams, and/or parts of your body.	❏	❏
11) To get feedback only when you have screwed up.	❏	❏

It's normal around here . . .	*Yes*	*No*

12) To receive more attention when you are down, ill, discouraged, saddened, and otherwise mired in the "Slough of Despond" than when you arrive at work ready to take on the world, jumping up and down with enthusiasm, urging fellow employees to "soar with the eagles" and accomplish great things today, etc. ❑ ❑

13) To tolerate or even ignore the potential harm of advertising during sports programming that promotes youthful drinking (eg, the use by Miller and Budweiser of athletic heroes depicted in bars having exuberant good times guzzling the sponsor's products). ❑ ❑

14) To not give priority to quality of life issues, such as protecting the environment, having fun in life, enjoying and taking pride in work, experiencing spiritual growth, and reaching out to others. ❑ ❑

© 1985 Donald B Ardell. Campus Wellness Center, University of Central Florida, Orlando FL 32816. Write Dr Ardell for permission to reproduce this test on a large scale basis or to include it in another publication.

TRAINER'S NOTES

©1994 Whole Person Press 210 W Michigan Duluth MN 55802   (800) 247-6789

81 PATHOLOGY OF NORMALCY

This satirical reading highlights the absurdity of powerful cultural norms that are antithetical to lifelong well-being.

GOALS

To help participants recognize how cultural norms work against the wellness lifestyle.

TIME FRAME

5 minutes

PROCESS

1) The trainer introduces the reading with some brief comments on the concept of "normalcy."

   ● It is human nature to want to be "normal"—to fit in with the people around us.

   ● Every group to which we belong has developed powerful norms that shape the behavior of its members. This is true for a family—it's also true for a society.

   ● The idea of "normal" influences our health-related behavior, too.

2) The trainer reads **The Pathology of Normalcy** essay.

3) Participants are invited to share their reactions and "confess" which points in the story hit home for them.

Submitted by Earl Hipp

©1994 Whole Person Press 210 W Michigan Duluth MN 55802   (800) 247-6789

THE PATHOLOGY OF NORMALCY by Earl Hipp

In our culture it is normal to eat when we're not hungry, to be overweight, to be overfat, to always take the elevator, and to drive around in the parking lot for five minutes to avoid a one minute walk. In fact, in our culture most people don't ever move faster than a walk unless it is absolutely necessary. Many normals prefer to watch others being physically active, while they sit and consume large quantities of saturated fat, salt, sugar and mood altering chemicals.

To be normal in our culture is to eat and drink a broad variety of chemicals, some of which cause disease in laboratory animals. Many normals do not enjoy food that doesn't taste like salt, and will often salt a whole meal before eating. It is also common for normals to reward their children's positive behaviors with massive doses of concentrated sugars.

Many normals are addicted to a brown, bitter tasting water that makes them feel anxious. To obscure the bitterness of this beverage, many will add saturated fat and sugar. Some normals inhale the smoke and tar of burning leaves, fully conscious of the fact that this behavior will shorten their lives, and the lives of those around them, by many years.

For two or three hours a day, normals will stare blankly at a small screen showing images of violence, artificial humor and unhealthy lifestyle behaviors. It is common that human interaction in many normal homes is confined to 60 second intervals between 15 minute periods of staring blankly at the small screen. On this same screen, before going to bed, normals will absorb a half hour of all the bad news that happened in their community and the world, and then read it all again the next morning in the newspaper to start the day.

Normals never really relax because they don't know how. It is considered normal in our culture to be occupied or preoccupied for all of your waking hours. Those who slow down are considered daydreamers and are invited to feel non-productive. This pace of living guarantees a high degree of stress for the normal person. Because of unmanaged stress, it is common for many normals to dramatically alter their mood with chemicals, and then drive two tons of metal at high speed, believing they are competent.

Because of this stress in their lives, it is difficult for normals to be playful. To avoid this stress, many normal individuals have adapted to a high degree of routine in their lives and do not willingly invite new challenges. In fact, many normals do not expect to experience joy or contentment on any regular basis, and go through life just getting by.

©1994 Whole Person Press 210 W Michigan Duluth MN 55802   (800) 247-6789

It is common for normals to have many acquaintances but few intimate friends. They are products of the "go it alone, be tough, don't show your pain" pioneer spirit of their forebears which invites them to not be real in their relationships and to feel cut off from others.

Normals do not expect their work life to be a lot of fun or extremely challenging after the first few years. For most, work is what they do for money and "The Benefits." Normals believe someone else will fix things that go wrong. For example, if they get sick or injured as a result of their lifestyle choices, medical science will repair them and their employer will be responsible for the costs. They also feel that if they vote once a year the world will be okay.

Normals do not know much of Health and Well-being or how to create those conditions. So when they do try to change their living habits, they start out enthusiastically—but most often fail. After a few attempts, most normals quit trying and resign themselves to the way they are.

All normals surround themselves with other normals who have similar values and behaviors. These people offer support to the normal person and help them to resist any significant change in their living habits. As a result of this support, normal people continue to be and feel normal.

*Because of the foregoing, normals in our culture miss out on much of the vitality, personal growth, joy and contentment they are capable of experiencing, and they die two to ten years before they have to. **All of this is normal in our culture.***

© 1986, Earl Hipp. All rights reserved.

82 WELL CARDS

Participants interpret wellness-oriented messages that they draw from a deck of cards and examine the implications for creating healthier lifestyles.

GOALS

To assess current lifestyle habits based on a wide variety of wellness messages.

To expand positive wellness attitudes and behaviors.

GROUP SIZE

Any size group is appropriate; also works well with individuals.

TIME REQUIRED

30–45 minutes

MATERIALS

A **Well Card** deck of **Wellness Messages** for each small group (to be prepared by the trainer ahead of time).

PROCESS

☞ *This exercise is more fun if each small group of 3–5 people has its own set of **Well Cards** prior to the session. Copy the **Well Card Messages** onto index cards or photocopy a set of pages for each group and cut them up in advance.*

1) The trainer introduces the activity with these comments:
   - Wellness-oriented quotations, quips and messages offer us a valuable source of ideas to examine and apply to our lifestyle attitudes and activities.
   - The wellness statements in the **Well Card** deck we will be using can prompt us to review our present lifestyle, but it remains a personal responsibility for each of us to implement necessary and profitable changes.

2) The trainer divides participants into groups of 3–5 members. He gives each group a **Well Card** deck and describes the process groups will use.
   - ➤ The **Well Cards** should be shuffled and placed in a stack face down for drawing.

©1994 Whole Person Press 210 W Michigan Duluth MN 55802   (800) 247-6789

➤ Participants will take turns drawing **Well Cards**.

➤ The first person draws a card, reads the wellness message, and comments on the meaning and significance of the statement for her personal life.

➤ As soon as she has shared her reactions, other group members are encouraged to add their views and experiences concerning the **Well Card** statement.

➤ The next person draws a new **Well Card** and follows the same procedure.

➤ You will have about *15 minutes* to explore as many cards as you wish. Don't rush—the idea is to explore the issues raised by the wellness messages, rather than finish the deck. Try to pace yourselves so that everyone has a chance to draw at least two cards.

3) After about 15 minutes, the trainer reassembles participants into one large group and asks those who wish to read the card they found most meaningful and to share with the group what lifestyle alterations this card suggested to them. The trainer leads a discussion about wellness attitudes and behaviors based on the group's comments.

VARIATIONS

■ Participants could be provided with blank index cards and invited to record and share additional wellness messages that they have found helpful. New entries for all wellness dimensions (physical, social, emotional, etc) should be encouraged.

■ Participants can use the **Well Cards** privately, recording notes and sorting out statements with personal significance.

Submitted by Kent Beeler.

©1994 Whole Person Press 210 W Michigan Duluth MN 55802   (800) 247-6789

WELL-CARD MESSAGES 1

Health is free, illness costs money. Safety is free, accidents are painful.	Beginning is winning.
The thrill of victory, the agony of defeat.	You alone can be well, but you can't be well alone. — Donald A Tubesing —
Your body is apt to be your autobiography.	Laughter is the music of the soul; relaxation is the health of the soul.
It is not so much we die; we kill ourselves.	No pain, no gain. Train, don't strain. No guts, no glory!
Your body is a Rolls Royce and is to be treated like one.	There are no simple solutions, only intelligent choices.
Wellness is the loving acceptance of yourself. — John W Travis —	The first wealth is health. — Ralph Waldo Emerson —
Every day think a beautiful thought, say a beautiful word and do a beautiful thing.	You are what you eat — so don't eat anything white! (salt, sugar, wonderbread)

WELL-CARD MESSAGES 2

Use it or lose it.	We know more about the service record of our car than our own health.
Not each of us can be a champion, but each of us can be a winner.	We keep a more complete health record for our pets than for ourselves.
Each patient carries his doctor inside him. — Albert Schweitzer —	People expect too much of medicine, too little of themselves.
Body, mind and soul are inextricably woven together and whatever helps or hurts one of these three sides of the whole man helps or hurts the other two. — Paul Dudley White —	Going on a diet suggests you will go off it.
Eat like a king at breakfast, a prince at lunch, a pauper at dinner.	Whatever you conceive and believe, you can achieve.
Don't sweat the small stuff— It's all small stuff!	What you eat in private shows in public. Once on the lips, forever on the hips
As a result of the wellness movement there are more smiles, fewer complaints, larger hearts, smaller doctor bills, and more satisfied lives. — Don Kemper —	To ward off disease or recover, men as a rule find it easier to depend upon healers than to attempt the more difficult task of living wisely. — Rene DuBois —

©1994 Whole Person Press 210 W Michigan Duluth MN 55802   (800) 247-6789

TRAINER'S NOTES

83 HEALTH LIFELINES

In this multi-stage exercise, participants draw their health lifelines, examining the patterns and critical incidents along the way. After writing autobiographical statements and "telling their stories," participants project their lifelines of well-being into the future.

GOALS

To explore and affirm personal uniqueness.

To outline a wellness history, identifying the critical incidents and lifelong health patterns that have shaped well-being.

To encourage the sharing of "personal stories" as a way of making positive contact with others.

To stimulate self-responsibility and "taking charge" of overall life direction and the quality of well-being.

GROUP SIZE

Unlimited; also appropriate for use with individuals or family units.

TIME FRAME

75–90 minutes

MATERIALS NEEDED

My Well-Being Lifeline worksheets and blank paper for each participant.

PROCESS

1) The trainer introduces the lifeline concept, highlighting some or all of these points:
   - **Every life has a line.** We move chronologically through time—a steady, regular progression of life experiences, each connected one to the other.
   - Sometimes we may feel that our lifeline is moving in a positive direction, sometimes it seems more negative. Often it is mixed—a bit of both. Always, however, **we live at the "end of the line,"** continually drawing the extension of our lifeline as the minutes, hours and days of our lives accumulate.

©1994 Whole Person Press 210 W Michigan Duluth MN 55802   (800) 247-6789

- **Life is composed of predictable patterns**, sudden turns and twists and various ups and downs, which when inter-connected over time form the fabric of our personal history, lay the foundation of our present, and suggest the possibilities for our future.

- Although many people share similar experiences, the subtle nuances of this history make each of us truly unique.

- **Wellness is a life-long process** of seeking to maintain our sense of well-being and to maximize the quality of our lives. We are always changing and adjusting our personal habits; always in the process of discovering both our potentials and our limitations; always making choices and commitments in light of our values and priorities.

- In order to plan for wellness, we must begin by examining our **wellness history** ("How did I get to where I am now?") and our current wellness status ("Where am I now?"). Only then can we make meaningful plans for maintaining—and, if necessary, regaining—our overall well-being.

2) The trainer supplies each participant with a copy of the **My Well-Being Lifeline** worksheet. Participants are instructed to draw a vertical line down the page at their current age.

3) The trainer asks participants to draw their well-being lifeline in the top part of their worksheet, using some or all of the guidelines outlined below:

➤ Reflect for a minute or two on your own history of well-being—from the whole person perspective.

➤ How has your physical, mental and spiritual health unfolded over the years?

➤ Have there been periods when you felt particularly healthy—or particularly "unwell"—in any of these dimensions?

➤ What about your overall sense of well-being over time?

➤ Draw a simple well-being lifeline from your birth to your current age, indicating as accurately as you can the "ups" and "downs" and "dramatic twists" you have experienced.

➤ Next embellish the line with words and images that help you recall what was going on in your life at various ages and stages.

➤ Jot down important traumas and triumphs. Recall significant changes and relationships.

➤ Pay particular attention to turning points when your line changed direction, as well as to the extremes, when your line was at its highest and lowest points.

> Spend about 5 minutes drawing and outlining the significant events of your whole person health history.

4) The trainer invites participants to explore some of the critical segments of their **Well-Being Lifeline** in more depth, using the process outlined below:

☞ *Allow enough time (3–4 minutes) for participants to reflect on each critical incident or measure.*

> Recall one or more *significant events* in your life, related to your overall well-being. *Write* them on the bottom half of your worksheet, below the approximate age when each event(s) occurred.

  ➤ Take a few minutes to make notes about these critical incidents. Bring the events to life once again in your mind and jot down the important details.

  ➤ What happened? How were you feeling? What changed? How did it begin? How did it end? Was it resolved? How was it resolved?

> *Draw an arrow* pointing to the time in your life that was the *most critical period* for your well-being.

  ➤ Make notes about the critical nature of this period.

  ➤ What was on the line? What was challenged? What strengths did you discover? What limitations? What helped you through it all?

> *Circle* the spot on your lifeline where you received your *most critical insight* about yourself and your well-being.

  ➤ Then record your reflections about this insight at the bottom of the worksheet.

  ➤ What did you discover? How did you come to this realization? What difference has it made in your daily life?

> Most people have received *significant support* from one or two key people at turning points in their lives. List the one or two people whose support at critical times has had a great positive impact on your well-being.

  ➤ Write down some details of this experience.

  ➤ When in your life did it occur? Who supported you? How? What difference did it make for your well-being? Why was this support so critical? So special?

5) The trainer distributes blank paper to everyone and explains the next step in the process—writing a brief well-being autobiography.

➤ Look over your drawing and notes on the worksheet. What patterns do you see? What continuity? What discontinuity? What has the flow of your life been like?

➤ Write a one page autobiography summarizing the quality of your life and well-being from birth to the present. Include all the insights and observations you can glean from the data on your **Lifeline** worksheet.

> You will have about ten minutes to write.

> Use whatever style comes naturally. Don't worry about grammar or spelling—this is for you, not your English teacher!

☞ *Some participants will record a chronological history ("I was born and then . . . and then . . . and then . . ."). Others may choose to highlight just the patterns, major transitions and normal rhythms of their lives. Each may approach this task in whatever way they like. Do encourage them, however, to highlight the factors in their history—both the joys and the pains—that add to their personal uniqueness.*

6) Participants gather in small discussion groups for "storytelling". For this the trainer divides participants into groups of 4 or 5 people, or utilizes previously established sharing units.

➤ Take 4 minutes each for telling your personal story.

➤ Begin by reading your autobiography, then embellishing it as you choose with incidents and examples from your **Well-Being Lifeline**.

The trainer keeps time and every 4 minutes directs the groups to begin listening to the stories of the next group member.

☞ *Remind people to listen to each other. They are not to pry for information which is not offered; nor are they to try to fix anything, to confront anyone, to give feedback, or to have pity on anyone. They are rather to listen and to appreciate the special uniqueness of each person's well-being as they are given the gift of hearing it.*

7) After all participants have had the opportunity to share part of their "story," the trainer instructs the small groups to discuss the nature and qualities of wellness exhibited by their group's life stories and identify the various forms of well-being present in their group. (5 minutes)

8) The trainer interrupts and asks groups to finish up their story-telling. After a minute or two, he asks participants to turn once again to their personal **Well-Being Lifeline** worksheet.

➤ This time focus on the future. Draw your line ten years into the future—depicting your well-being as you would like to see it develop over that time period.

9) The trainer asks participants the following questions one at a time, suggesting they write their answers on the worksheet (if there is space) or on blank paper. (1–2 minutes each)

➤ What is the meaning of the line you have drawn? (What will happen? How will you feel? Body, mind and spirit? What will your wellness be like?)

➤ What are the three most important things you must do on your own behalf to ensure that your well-being lifeline unfolds as you have drawn it?

➤ When and how are you willing to take these steps for yourself?

10) Participants briefly share with their small group this vision of their future well-being and their self-care resolutions for making the vision come true. (5 minutes)

11) The trainer reconvenes the entire group and solicits observations and insights about personal well-being that occurred to participants during this exercise.

VARIATION

■ This extended sequence of reflection and sharing could be shortened by cutting one or more steps. The depth and impact of the process would be correspondingly reduced.

■ If time is limited, the trainer would be advised to cut part of the process rather than to rush through it all. Participants will find it difficult and frustrating to be asked to reflect on the totality of their life "in a hurry."

TRAINER'S NOTES

©1994 Whole Person Press 210 W Michigan Duluth MN 55802   (800) 247-6789

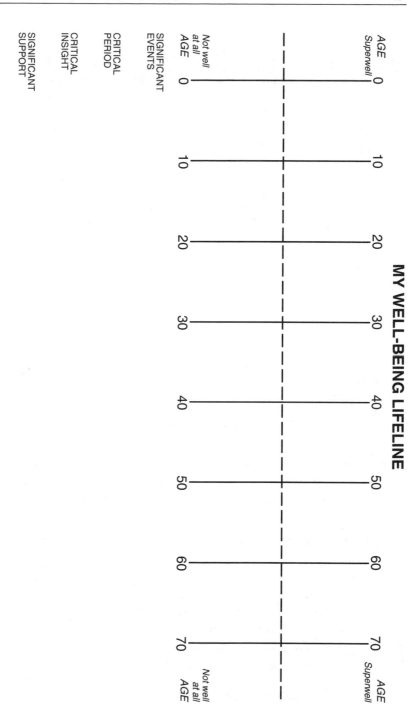

MY WELL-BEING LIFELINE

AGE Superwell

AGE Not well at all

AGE Superwell

AGE Not well at all

SIGNIFICANT EVENTS / AGE

CRITICAL PERIOD

CRITICAL INSIGHT

SIGNIFICANT SUPPORT

©1994 Whole Person Press 210 W Michigan Duluth MN 55802   (800) 247-6789

84 STAND UP AND BE COUNTED

In this wellness habit quiz, participants graphically answer ten lifestyle questions with their feet—moving from one side of the room to the other to demonstrate their responses.

GOALS

To assess personal wellness lifestyle habits.

To demonstrate that health is affected by many varied choices.

To make the variations in personal styles graphically visible.

GROUP SIZE

Unlimited; but must have space to move from one side of the room to the other.

TIME FRAME

15–20 minutes

PROCESS

1) The trainer introduces the exercise by pointing out that our health is affected both positively and negatively by the many varied choices we make each day.

2) The trainer announces that he will lead the group through a ten-item lifestyle assessment questionnaire. However, rather than answer the questions on paper, participants will "write" their answers with their feet!

3) The trainer designates one wall of the room as the "yes" response side, and the opposite wall for the "no" response.

   Participants are instructed to stand, listen to the first question and then indicate their answer by moving toward the appropriate wall. Once they have arrived at the wall, they are to turn back to the room and face the participants on the opposite wall.

   ☞ *Announce to the group that you will participate in this exercise by moving from one wall to the other, as well! If you are using a microphone, be sure the cord is long enough so that you can stand up and be counted, too!*

©1994 Whole Person Press 210 W Michigan Duluth MN 55802   (800) 247-6789

4) The trainer asks the first question:

☞ *Be sure to repeat which wall is "yes" and which is "no" (or you may want to post newsprint signs).*

If, on any question, some participants stay in the middle of the room, not sure which way to go, you may give them permission to stay there if, and only if, they physically waver back and forth. They must keep moving back and forth, acting out their indecision in order to be allowed to stay in the middle. If they want to stop this vacillating they must move to one of the walls!

➤ **Question #1: I always get enough sleep to get up refreshed in the morning.** Yes or no? Consider your answer and then at the signal move as rapidly as possible toward one wall or the other.

The trainer gives the signal—MOVE—and participants go to the appropriate wall.

☞ *You may want to encourage participants to look at the eyeballs of the people on the opposite wall and decide whether they answered truthfully!*

5) The trainer asks the remaining questions, instructing participants to move to the appropriate wall in response to each question.

☞ *Make whatever observations occur to you as you ask the questions and as people move themselves from one side of the room to the other. The movement will vary from question to question and, if you keep the pace rapid, the momentum will build.*

➤ **Question #2: I always wear my seat belt when in a moving vehicle.** Yes or no? MOVE!

☞ *If the group is in a playful mood, this is an opportunity to joke about the people who always use their seat belts—identify them as compulsives or pessimists!*

➤ **Question #3: I am within 5 pounds of the normal weight standard for my height and build.** Yes or no? MOVE!

☞ *After people move you may want to say something like, "This is probably the only item where we can all do some reality testing!" Ask how many people would have been on the other side of the room 5 years ago.*

➤ **Question #4: I don't smoke cigarettes—or anything else!** Yes or no? MOVE!

☞ *You may get some chuckles—and some people who change direction! —if you pause before saying, "or anything else!" Ask how many people would have been on the other side 5 years ago.*

➤ **Question #5: I know how to measure my own blood pressure.** Yes or no? MOVE!

☞ *Challenge those who answered "no" to look over the "yes" group and identify someone to ask to teach them how to take their own blood pressure!*

➤ **Question #6: I know how to measure my resting heart rate.** Yes or no? MOVE!

☞ *Ask the "yes" side of the room to demonstrate the proper technique, and comment on how well they do. Instruct all participants to take their own pulse before moving on to the next question. Keep time for them as a group.*

➤ **Question #7: My resting heart rate is 60 beats per minute or less.** Yes or no? MOVE!

☞ *This is a tougher question! There won't be many people left on the "yes" side, especially if you ask them to consider their current heart rate!*

➤ **Question #8: I know and use three methods for reducing stress and tension without using alcohol or other drugs.** Yes or no? MOVE!

☞ *The "other drugs" may turn some people in their tracks— especially if caffeine and sugar are included.*

➤ **Question #9: On the average I drink less than four units of alcohol per week.** Yes or no? MOVE!

☞ *One unit equals one shot hard liquor, one beer or six ounces of wine. You may alter the number of units as you see fit, but more than seven per week (one a day) should definitely be a "no" response!*

➤ **Question #10: I have three people in my life with whom I can share my inner most fears and triumphs.** Yes or no? MOVE!

☞ *You may turn to those on the "no" side and say, "Go it alone if you like, but I've just cancelled your health insurance! Data shows that you 'tough-it-out-by-yourself-hard-core-loners' are simply too great a risk!"*

6) The trainer reconvenes the group and inquires about participants' scores.

✔ Did anyone answer "yes" to all 10 questions?

☞ *You may want to joke, "If there's a perfect 10 here, you ought to be leading this group!"*

✔ How many people had 9 "yes" answers?

☞ *There may be a few. Congratulate them warmly.*

✔ What about 8 "yes" answers? How many with 7? Six?

☞ *At the number that corresponds to your personal score on the test, you should raise your hand along with the others.*

✔ I don't want to embarrass anyone too much, but how many people scored 5 or less on this little quiz?

☞ *Usually a third to a half of the audience will fall in this group. You may want to challenge them by saying, "When I was in school 50% or less on an exam meant you flunked! Unfortunately, the exam here is your life! Fortunately, it's not too late to change your answers. With a score of 5 or less you have the opportunity to experiment with several new ways of living that can enhance your health."*

7) The trainer asks participants to share their observations and insights about the test and their self-care habits. After several people have shared, the trainer issues a final challenge:

● We all engage in some behaviors that promote health and some that deplete our health. **No one is totally self-destructive and no one is perfect!**

● If you are interested in changing your answers to any of these questions you will need to alter the way you live. The remainder of this learning experience will offer you the opportunity to **assess what lifestyle changes you would like to make** and teach you some skills to implement them.

8) The trainer closes the exercise on a humorous note:

● The exercise you have participated in during the last few minutes has helped you burn off an additional 13 calories (one Wheat Thin cracker, one thimble of beer, or one M & M). But the laughter and interaction you have shared appears to have more than doubled your vitality!

©1994 Whole Person Press 210 W Michigan Duluth MN 55802   (800) 247-6789

VARIATIONS

■ This process of "answering with your feet" can be used with any set of questions about personal lifestyle which are likely to be answered differently by different people (eg, 10 questions on how you manage stress, or your nutrition habits, or your support network). Adjust the list of questions to the objectives of your session, or personalize the questions to the specific behavior patterns and temptations of the group you're working with.

■ If time limitations or the room size do not permit movement from wall to wall, participants can be instructed to count their "yes" responses on their fingers. However, this compromise will cut the physical movement, and the laughter from the process and thus diminish the energy and vitality that can be generated.

TRAINER'S NOTES

Submitted by Bill Hettler.

©1994 Whole Person Press 210 W Michigan Duluth MN 55802   (800) 247-6789

Self-Care
Strategies

85 AUTO/BODY CHECKUP

This quick health assessment uses the metaphor of the automobile to compare the maintenance required for our cars to the care required for our own well-being.

GOALS

To help assess personal wellness style.

To promote positive attitudes toward self-care and to stimulate the sharing of these attitudes.

GROUP SIZE

Unlimited.

TIME FRAME

15–20 minutes

MATERIALS NEEDED

One copy of **The Auto/Body Checkup** form and **Observations** worksheet for each participant.

PROCESS

1) The trainer introduces the exercise by pointing out the similarities between the maintenance of an automobile and the self-care required to maintain our personal well-being.

   - It is possible to drive both our cars and our bodies as fast and as far as possible until they quit on us. Then we haul them in for repair with the instructions, "Get this (auto/body) back on the road as soon as possible."

   - However, both cars and people work better over the long run when they receive regular refueling and appropriate preventive maintenance.

   - People develop patterns of caring for their cars. They also develop a personal style of self-care.

2) The trainer distributes **The Auto/Body Checkup** form and **Observations** worksheet to participants. She instructs them first to complete the

©1994 Whole Person Press 210 W Michigan Duluth MN 55802   (800) 247-6789

Checkup, paying particular attention to their attitudes regarding regular maintenance of both their cars and their bodies.

☞ *The **Auto/Body Checkup** form is basically a consciousness raising tool. It is meant to stimulate discussion, not assess behavior. Participant insights will be recorded on the **Observations** worksheet.*

Once everyone has finished the checklist, the trainer invites participants to reflect on their auto- and self-care patterns, using the **Observations** worksheet.

3) The trainer divides participants into groups of 3–4 persons each and invites them to share the insights they discovered while completing the worksheets.

☞ *Encourage people in their sharing to pay particular attention to any surprising observations that occurred to them.*

4) The trainer reconvenes the entire group and solicits comments from participants.

VARIATIONS

■ Prior to distributing the worksheet, the trainer could lead participants through a guided visualization in which they create a mental picture of their "dream car"—including the make, the model, the year, the accessories, the color, the interior, etc.

■ Participants could also be helped to visualize their "dream body"— including size, looks, capabilities, interior and exterior design and functioning, etc. Following the completion of the worksheet, participants may be asked to reflect on whether their current self-care habits are likely to create for them the body of their dreams.

☞ *Both of these variations can be used effectively with teenagers.*

Submitted by Martha Belknap

TRAINER'S NOTES

AUTO/BODY CHECKUP, Part 1

MY CAR		MY BODY
The **fuel** I need for my car is: ❑ regular ❑ lead free ❑ diesel ❑ supreme	FUEL	The **fuels** I need for my body are: ❑ fresh fruit/juices ❑ dairy products ❑ nuts/seeds ❑ whole grain cereals ❑ fresh vegetables ❑ meat/fish/poultry/eggs
My car runs best when I keep the **fluids** clean, so I regularly check and change: ❑ oil ❑ radiator level ❑ brake fluid ❑ windshield washer fluid ❑ power steering	FLUIDS	My body runs best when I keep **the blood clean,** so I need to check my intake of: ❑ sugar ❑ salt ❑ fats ❑ chemicals ❑ medications
I check the **air** in my: ❑ tires ❑ air cleaner (filter)	AIR	I check the **air in my lungs.** I need to regulate the intake of: ❑ smoke ❑ smog ❑ fumes ❑ dust ❑ nicotine ❑ pollen ❑ toxins
Additives in my car effect its effieciency. I regularly use: ❑ oil additives ❑ gas additives	ADDITIVES	**Additives** can effect my nervous system. I need to regulate the intake of: ❑ caffeine ❑ alcohol ❑ stimulants ❑ drugs

AUTO/BODY CHECKUP, Part 2

MY CAR		MY BODY
BODY WORK		
To improve its **appearance** my car needs: ❑ washing ❑ waxing ❑ vacuuming ❑ body repairs (dents/rusting) ❑ personal decorations for the special touch		To improve **my appearance**, I need to work on my: ❑ skin/hair/neck ❑ teeth ❑ weight ❑ posture ❑ breath/body odor ❑ personal sparkle and style
MAINTENANCE		
My car engine needs a **regular tune-up.** I need to check: ❑ points ❑ plugs ❑ condenser ❑ filters ❑ hoses ❑ belts ❑ tires ❑ timing ❑ alignment		My body needs **regular checkups** as well as **rest and activity.** I need to provide for: ❑ sleep/relaxation ❑ physical contact/sex ❑ solitude ❑ mental stimulation ❑ regular medical checkup ❑ humor/fun ❑ regular dental checkup ❑ creative expressions ❑ stretching/exercise ❑ centering alignment ❑ companionship/love
POWER		
In order to get going, my car needs a good **electrical system.** I need to check: ❑ ignition ❑ battery ❑ alternator ❑ voltage regulator		In order to get going, my body/mind needs a **good belief system.** I need to check: ❑ self concept ❑ attitudes ❑ expectations ❑ goals ❑ faith
HANDLING		
In order to drive my car safely, I need to: ❑ go easy ❑ limit my speed ❑ look ahead		To run my life safely and efficiently, I need to: ❑ keep myself in control ❑ pace myself ❑ plan ahead

©1994 Whole Person Press 210 W Michigan Duluth MN 55802   (800) 247-6789

OBSERVATIONS

In looking over the maintenance requirements for my car and observing how carefully I attend to them—I would say my style of caring for my car is:

In looking over the maintenance requirements for my body and observing my habits of caring for (or not caring for) myself—I would say my style of taking care of my body is:

In comparing these two styles, I would say that:

_____ I care for my car and my body in about the same pattern.

_____ I care for my car better than I care for my body.

_____ I care for my body better than I care for my car.

I believe that _____ my body or _____ my car is most important to my long range well-being.

In the future, I would like to take better care of myself by regularly doing the following:

Final thoughts/comments:

86 CHEMICAL INDEPENDENCE

In this exercise, participants examine the reasons for—and the results of—alcohol use in our society. They then personalize the issue by analyzing their own use patterns.

GOALS

To raise consciousness about the patterns of alcohol use in this society.

To give participants the opportunity to think through their own current relationship with alcohol.

GROUP SIZE

Since participants are divided into three working groups, this exercise works best with 12–30 people. It can be adapted, however, for use with larger groups.

TIME FRAME

25–35 minutes

MATERIALS NEEDED

One copy of the **Alcohol Use Profile** worksheet for each participant.

PROCESS

1) The trainer introduces the subject of this exercise, alcohol use, pointing out that the purpose of this process is to examine the attitudes and use patterns of society, as well as the personal styles and beliefs of each participant.

   ☞ *To avoid appearing judgmental, you may want to point out that you're not going to point fingers at anyone. Rather, you will ask two basic questions, "What do we do?" and "Does what we do make sense?"*

2) The trainer divides participants into three groups and gives instructions.
   ➤ Group #1 should brainstorm a list of *reasons why people drink.*
   ➤ Group #2 should develop a list of *problems associated with alcohol misuse and abuse.*
   ➤ Group #3 should generate a list of *reasons for not drinking.*
   (5-8 minutes)

©1994 Whole Person Press 210 W Michigan Duluth MN 55802   (800) 247-6789

☞ *Give a warning after 5 minutes and then allow 2 more minutes.*

3) The trainer reassembles the participants. Group #1 shares their list of *reasons why people drink*. The trainer summarizes the points on the blackboard as they are presented, listing them in one single vertical column on the left side of the board. Participants from the other groups are invited to add additional reasons that occur to them.

   After all ideas are recorded, the trainer asks the group to decide which reasons for using alcohol are primarily the result of peer pressure, and marks them with a star.

4) Group #2 summarizes the *problems associated with alcohol misuse and abuse* and the trainer records their ideas on the blackboard in a second vertical column, parallel to the first.

   Participants then look for connections between individual *reasons for drinking* and specific *problems that result.* The trainer draws connecting lines between associated pairs.

5) Group #3 shares their list of *reasons for not drinking,* which the trainer records in a third parallel column.

   The trainer then asks which *reasons for not drinking* could provide a corrective for the *problems that result from drinking.* Lines are again drawn between columns to show whatever connections are suggested.

6) The trainer observes that many of the items in all three lists relate to social occasions and friendships. She asks the group to generate a list of all the occasions where people drink.

   The trainer raises the following questions for discussion.

   ✔ Can we make a decision not to drink and still have friends? The same friends? Will they relate in the same way?

   ✔ If not, why not?

   ✔ How much do our friendships and our good times revolve around alcohol use?

7) The trainer distributes a copy of the **Alcohol Use Profile** to each participant, and instructs them to complete the first half of the worksheet—the twelve question quiz—and to total their "yes" answers.

8) The trainer presents a rough scoring guideline for the quiz and invites participants to interpret their own scores. She notes that the significance of the test lies not in the score, but in the patterns it reveals.

©1994 Whole Person Press 210 W Michigan Duluth MN 55802   (800) 247-6789

- **0-2 "yes" responses** probably indicates that alcohol use is not currently a problem for you. Don't be smug, but do keep up the healthy pattern.

- **3-6 "yes" responses** indicates that you are not really independent of alcohol at this point in your life. It's likely that your well-being is in some way negatively affected by your alcohol use patterns. You might want to rethink your current habits.

- **7-12 "yes" responses** indicates that your use of, and dependence upon, alcohol has reached a dangerous level in your life. You would be wise to commit yourself to cutting back! And, if you find after some attempt to curtail your use of alcohol that you have not been successful, you would do yourself, your family and friends a favor by asking someone to help you regain control. Don't wait until you're in deep trouble! Find out what's going on inside you and take steps to change your style **Now!**

- This quiz is not perfect, nor is the scoring system "scientific." It does, however, invite each of us to examine our own patterns of alcohol use. So, the best scoring standard is your own reaction to your answers. "How do you feel about the patterns you see?"

9) The trainer asks participants to complete the **Analysis and Reflection** section of the worksheet.

VARIATION

- As written, this exercise focuses solely on alcohol use. The process could be just as applicable to an analysis and discussion of patterns for using any addictive substance: food, tobacco, caffeine, chocolate, marijuana, cocaine, etc.

*The process for this exercise was submitted by Sandy Queen. The **Alcohol Use Profile** was submitted by Merrill Kempfert.*

©1994 Whole Person Press 210 W Michigan Duluth MN 55802   (800) 247-6789

ALCOHOL USE PROFILE

1) Do you drink to deal with stress, to get away   Y   N
   from the press of responsibilities or to relax?

2) Do you sometimes drink because everyone   Y   N
   else is or "simply because it's available"?

3) Has drinking caused you any difficulty with   Y   N
   family or friends, or at work?

4) Do you ever drive after drinking to the degree   Y   N
   that you would be nervous if stopped by the
   police and asked to take a Breathalyzer test?

5) Do you ever misrepresent or cover up the   Y   N
   amount that you drink?

6) Do you, at times, find it a struggle to have only   Y   N
   1 or 2 drinks and then stop?

7) Do you sometimes drink more than you plan   Y   N
   or think you should?

8) Does it annoy you if someone hints that you   Y   N
   drink too much?

9) Do you drink differently (more, faster, more   Y   N
   potent drinks) than your companions?

10) Have you ever felt proud of the amount you   Y   N
    could consume and not show it?

11) Do you get pleasure from the feeling you   Y   N
    experience when alcohol starts to affect you?

12) Do you ever feel guilty about your drinking?   Y   N

ANALYSIS AND REFLECTION

What does the instructor's scoring system say about your score?

What patterns of alcohol use do you see in your life these days?

How are your alcohol use patterns different now than they were five years ago?

How do you feel about these patterns?

What problems does your current use of alcohol cause you?

Do you want to make any changes? If so, what?

©1994 Whole Person Press 210 W Michigan Duluth MN 55802   (800) 247-6789

87 CONSCIOUSNESS-RAISING DIET

Participants use Dr Christopher's memorable questions to raise their consciousness about attitudes toward eating.

GOALS

To examine reasons for food choices and eating patterns.

To experiment with healthy standards for determining what and when to eat.

GROUP SIZE

Unlimited; also works well with individuals.

TIME FRAME

10–15 minutes

PROCESS

1) The trainer introduces the exercise with a brief synopsis of factors that influence eating patterns.

   - During the 1970's most Americans bought into the popular philosophy that urged us, **"If it feels good, do it!"** Although we now realize how self-defeating that attitude can be, most of us have not fully adjusted our food choices.

   - People usually judge the quality and appropriateness of their food by asking three questions:
     - **Does it taste good?**
     - **Does it look good?**
     - **Does it smell good?**

     When the answer to these questions is "yes," we may eat without giving it another thought!

   - **Many people use taste as a justification for eating.** When asked, "Why did you eat that?," they respond, "It tasted good!" No wonder! We are deluged by food-related advertisements that promote food consumption based on taste, looks and smell (eg, "tastes great," "melts in your mouth," etc).

2) The trainer asks the group to generate a list of advertising slogans used to "sell" us on eating a variety of food products. The trainer lists all suggestions on the board, and leads the group in a short discussion on the motivation for eating underlying each of the phrases.

3) The trainer offers an alternative model for making decisions about what we eat—Dr Christopher's consciousness-raising diet questions.

   ● A wellness consciousness calls for us to ask two additional questions about our food.
      ○ **Do I need it?**
      ○ **Is it healthy for me?**

   ● If the answer to *Question #4* is "No, I don't need it," then we would be better off not eating—even if in abstract it could be healthy for us.

   ● If the answer to *Question #5* is "No, it's not healthy for me," then we would be better off finding something else to eat that will fill our need.

   ● If the answer to both *Questions #4* and *#5* is "Yes, I need it and it is good for me," then we should reflect once again on the first three questions and eat the best tasting, best smelling and best looking samples we can find.

4) The trainer asks participants to analyze their last meal (or their last snack—if it was a major event!) raising the five-eating related questions about each item they consumed. He suggests that participants pay particular attention to their answers to *Questions #4* and *#5*. What they would have consumed if they had taken their answers to these questions seriously.

5) The trainer challenges participants to apply at their next meal what they have learned in this exercise.

   ● For any item you consider eating, first stop and ask yourself *Questions #4* and *#5*: Do I need it? Is it healthy?

   ● Eat only those items for which you can answer "yes" to both questions.

   ● Note the difference these two consciousness-raising questions make in the quality and quantity of what you eat.

      ☞ *This exercise is particularly effective when used just prior to a meal. Participants may be asked to report on their eating behavior when they return from the meal.*

Submitted by Grant Christopher, MD

88 COUNTDOWN TO RELAXATION

In this quick and simple relaxation exercise participants learn to deepen their relaxation response. This whole person approach is particularly involving since it combines physical relaxation with visual and auditory stimuli.

GOALS

To demonstrate the effectiveness of using all three primary perceptual modalities (kinesthetic, visual and auditory) in a self-regulation exercise.

To teach a rapid, self-regulated method of deepening relaxation response.

GROUP SIZE

Unlimited; can be used individually as well as in group instruction and demonstration.

TIME FRAME

5–10 minutes

PROCESS

1) The trainer outlines the goals of this relaxation experience and invites participants to make themselves comfortable—find a relaxed, balanced posture (seated), loosen clothing, remove glasses, etc.

   ☞ *Be sure the atmosphere is conducive to relaxation—dim lighting, quiet, freedom from interruptions.*

2) The trainer guides participants through the **Countdown to Relaxation** exercise, using the script below.

3) The trainer waits for people to open their eyes and then invites participants to share their reactions and ideas for personal application of the **Countdown** process.

   After several people have shared, he closes the exercise with two final bits of information.

   ● With regular practice you will soon be able to condense this process from a 100-countdown to a 10-countdown. You will then be able to elicit the relaxation response quickly in most situations.

- This technique works especially well for falling asleep. Most people will enter sleep or very deep relaxation by the time the countdown is to the 50's.

  If you are still awake after two cycles of counting down from 100, you should try another relaxation technique.

TRAINER'S NOTES

Submitted by David X Swenson.

COUNTDOWN TO RELAXATION Script

Lean back and relax as comfortably as possible . . .
You may want to close your eyes as you take a deep breath and focus your attention inward . . .

Take another deep breath and quickly scan your body for tension. Whenever you notice any tightness, breathe into that area . . . And then release the tension as you exhale . . . You may even want to sigh as you let go of the tension that has stored up . . .

Take another deep breath and feel the tension drain away as you exhale . . .

☞ *Continue with deep breathing or another basic relaxation approach for a minute or two.*

Now I'd like you to imagine that you are in front of a large movie screen . . . Somewhat like a drive-in theatre . . .
Let the screen fill your entire visual field . . . As far as you look . . . up and down . . . left and right . . . the empty screen is all you can see.

Notice the color of the screen . . . Notice its texture . . .

Now allow the number "100" to appear on the screen . . .
Notice the shape . . . color . . . texture . . . Perhaps the sound of saying the number . . . Just notice and appreciate the presence of the number . . .

Let the number change from "100" to "99" . . .
Notice how it changes . . . Does it fall like a card? . . . disperse like a mist? . . . blink out? . . . melt or dissolve? . . . crumble into bits? . . . just change its form? . . .

Notice how the numbers are formed . . . rounded? . . . angular? . . . three dimensional? . . . Does the color change in some subtle way? . . .

At your own pace let the numbers continue to change . . .
Every few relaxing breaths the number can change . . .
Each time it changes you can relax even more deeply . . .

☞ *Give people about 3 minutes to countdown on their own before ending the exercise.*

Now it's time to stop counting . . . Just allow whatever number is on your screen to disappear and then return your attention to this room and this group . . . Take whatever time you need, knowing that when you open your eyes you will remain just as comfortable and deeply relaxed as you now feel.

89 FIT TO BE INTERVIEWED

In this between-session activity, participants interview people who regularly engage in an appealing physical fitness activity. It is designed to motivate participants toward an active personal fitness plan.

GOALS

To increase interest in beginning a personal fitness program.

To gain first-hand information about a sport, physical activity or exercise in which participants are willing to consider becoming involved.

GROUP SIZE

Described for small groups (6–15 people), easily adaptable for larger groups or individual use.

TIME FRAME

10 minutes for introductions; interviews can usually be conducted in 15–20 minutes; group follow-up discussion requires about 30 minutes.

MATERIALS NEEDED

One copy of the **Fit To Be Interviewed** form for each participant.

PROCESS

☞ *This exercise works best as a follow-up to a presentation on the health benefits of a regular exercise program.*

1) The trainer begins by asking participants to make a list of the people they know who value physical fitness and who engage in a regular exercise program. Beside each name they should note the different sports or activities that the person usually chooses for exercise (2 minutes).

2) The trainer announces that this activity is a homework assignment to be completed before the next session. He describes the purpose of the activity as outlined in the **Goals** and notes that the impact of the experience will be maximized if people choose to interview someone whose style of exercising is intriguing to them.

➤ Look over your list of people and exercise options and circle (or star) all the activities and sports that you find particularly interesting.

©1994 Whole Person Press 210 W Michigan Duluth MN 55802   (800) 247-6789

➤ Underline the names of people who would be good candidates for interviewing because they engage in interesting physical fitness activities.

3) The trainer distributes **Fit To Be Interviewed** forms and provides participants with general guidelines for conducting the interview.

➤ Select an interviewee who exercises a minimum of three times a week for at least 15–20 minutes each time. This person does not have to be a competitive athlete or a team member; individuals who participate at a recreational level are eligible.

➤ Arrange for a 15–20 minute interview with the candidate—this could be done by phone if necessary. Explain that you would like her or him to answer a series of brief questions designed to help you in setting up a similar fitness program.

➤ Record the candidate's answers on the **Fit To Be Interviewed** form.

➤ Immediately after the interview, take some time to consider your reactions by answering the questions in the **Interviewer's Debriefing** section of the form.

➤ Bring your completed forms to the next meeting.

☞ *Before adjourning be sure that all participants have more than one potential candidate in mind, in case they can't interview their top choice. It helps to have them pin this down in writing.*

4) Participants bring completed **Fit To Be Interviewed** forms to the next session. The trainer leads a discussion of the interview results. Participants share their immediate plans for beginning a physical activity or exercise routine.

VARIATIONS

■ With more than 15 people, divide into smaller groups (4–8 people) for the discussion and plan-sharing process in *Step 4*. The leaderless groups could meet concurrently or the trainer could meet separately with each group and facilitate the discussion.

■ Participants with an interest in similar areas of physical activities or exercises can meet together and discuss responses on their interview forms and share their personal plans for beginning a fitness plan.

Submitted by Kent Beeler.

TRAINER'S NOTES

FIT TO BE INTERVIEWED

Name of Interviewee _____ Age ___ Sex ___

1) What is the main fitness activity or sport you engage in?

2) How often do you do this each week? How many minutes/hours each time?

3) How long (months, years) have you been exercising like this?

4) Why did you begin?

5) What barriers did you have to overcome to get started? How did you deal with these obstacles?

6) What helps you to keep going with your fitness program?

7) What are the major benefits in maintaining a regular fitness schedule?

8) What are the most difficult aspects of keeping it up?

9) Do you plan to continue this fitness activity regularly? Why or why not?

10) Would you recommend your fitness activity for someone who is just beginning a physical fitness program? Why or why not?

11) What else would you like to add?

12) Thanks for your help! Keep up the great work!

©1994 Whole Person Press 210 W Michigan Duluth MN 55802   (800) 247-6789

INTERVIEWER'S DEBRIEFING

1) In this interview, what fitness ideas intrigued you most?

2) What did you learn that is applicable to your own life situation and fitness status?

3) What did you learn that could help you successfully embark on or continue a regular fitness program?

4) Based on this interview, what do you want to do about your own fitness program?

90 JOURNAL TO MUSIC

This exercise enhances participants' sense of well-being by helping them clarify vague and elusive feelings, images and personal goals. The process combines personal reflection and writing with listening to music.

GOALS

To enhance feeling-level reaction to life experiences by journal writing.

To encourage the use of music to bridge the gap between the language of physiology and the language of consciousness.

GROUP SIZE

Unlimited; more intense with groups of 8–10 people.

TIME FRAME

60–90 minutes

PHYSICAL SETTING

Informal, "homey" lounge area with sofas, comfortable chairs and clipboards is preferable to tables and chairs. Lighting should be dimmed. A quiet atmosphere without interruptions is essential. Fresh air is great—the session may be held outside or windows left open if the weather is nice.

MATERIALS NEEDED

Fine point colored markers, unlined paper; kleenex; tape recorder and preselected music (see guidelines at the end of the exercise).

PROCESS

1) The trainer welcomes the group and explains that this meeting may be different from others since the goal is to learn one specific skill—journaling—that participants will be experimenting with "on their own." He urges that no one be fooled by the apparent lack of action, since journaling can be an extremely powerful tool for stress management and health enhancement.

2) The trainer introduces the concept of journaling, covering some or all of the following points:

- **Journaling is a writing process** often confused with keeping a diary or record-keeping. Journaling is more than the simple logging of events. It promotes in-depth self-guided personal exploration.
- **The goal of journaling is the expressing on paper of our thoughts and feelings.** Often, writing down our images and feelings enhances our ability to sort out what is truly meaningful and assists us in gaining perspective on the behavioral changes we are trying to make. Since this process is private, we can be totally honest as we write.
- **Journaling makes tangible what is normally elusive.** Our thoughts and feelings become more concrete when we not only "think" them, but also write, read and respond to them. Writing also suggests a permanence through which commitment for change is enhanced.
- **Music can be combined with journaling to help us slow down and relax**—to become aware of our emotions and images that lie buried and unrecognized under our hectic schedules. Music also communicates in rhythms that evoke associations and feelings that are not otherwise readily accessible.
- Most people who keep journals periodically refer back to what they have written at an earlier time—so **dating journal entries is important.** If we document when we have experienced certain feelings or images, we can see over time the development of new attitudes and behavioral changes.

3) The trainer describes the process that will be used:
- ➤ Music and a brief relaxation experience will help everyone get settled down and centered.
- ➤ The next 20 minutes will be spent writing about some aspect of your life. What you write is for your eyes only, unless you choose to share it. There will be time at the end of the writing process for people to read aloud what they have written if they so desire, but there will be no pressure.
- ➤ The idea is to "go with the flow" of your thought pattern. Don't worry too much about what you are writing. Just get your pen or pencil moving across the page, recording the images that come to mind.
  - ➤ Spelling, grammar, vocabulary and sentence structure don't count here. You may have to write the same thing down over and over until a new thought comes. The goal is to take abstract, fleeting thoughts and make them concrete.

➤ Sometimes it helps to use different colored markers to high-light special feelings, to doodle, or to get unstuck. Occasionally sad, frightening or strange thoughts will come to mind and tears or laughter may well up in you. Terrific! You're in touch with something important. See if you can capture it in words.

4) The trainer asks if there are any questions about the process, noting that once the exercise begins it will be important for everyone to maintain silence.

5) When all questions are answered and participants are reassured, he leads them through a short relaxation routine (eg, closed eyes, deep breathing, mental surrender). (5 minutes)

6) The trainer turns on appropriate music (see Guidelines on p 75) and guides the group into music journaling.

➤ As the music begins allow yourself to "flow" with the music as much as possible, letting go of physical tension and allowing your mind to drift toward a significant aspect of your life that you would like to write about.

☞ *Reassure participants that it may take several minutes to get focused on a direction to pursue. Encourage them to take all the time they need. Wait a minute or two for people to get in the mood before the next instruction.*

➤ Once you have decided on an area to explore in depth, mentally massage that dimension of life and when you feel ready, open your eyes and start writing.

☞ *Once they start writing, remind participants to concentrate on their own experience, saying something like, "Eyes should be on your own journal as you write—avoid eye contact with others." As a facilitator, you are also a participant and should begin to journal yourself!*

7) After 15–20 minutes for writing, the trainer breaks the silence, inform-ing participants that they may continue writing, if they choose to, while the floor is opened for the second part of the journaling process— reading aloud. He describes the process and purpose of this part of the activity:

➤ Anyone may share what they have written by reading out loud as much of their journal entry as they care to—from a line or two to a major portion.

> ➤ This sharing is strictly confidential! What is seen and heard here must stay here.

> ➤ It is for the reader's benefit only. No questions or comments are permitted from other participants or from the leader.

> ➤ In fact, this step could be done just as effectively by reading to a tree, since the real value comes from seeing, saying and hearing the feelings that you have sorted out and expressed on paper. This "extra-sensory input" often enhances self-understanding.

> ➤ You may want to use a different colored pen to capture and jot in the margin any "aha" insights you experience during the reading.

After reassuring the group that it's fine not to share anything, the trainer announces that the floor will be open during the next 10 minutes for reading out loud. He explains that the silence is meant as an opportunity—not as a pressure.

☞ *The trainer needs to be comfortable with silence. Wait patiently for someone to start the sharing. Reduce pressure by sitting still and avoiding eye contact with participants. The time for reading can be extended if many people want to share what they have written.*

8) The trainer announces that the floor will close in two minutes and at the appropriate time summarizes the importance of reading as an essential component to the journaling process. He offers to answer questions from the group and comments on the journaling process—but not on the specific content read and shared by participants.

9) In closing, the trainer encourages participants to start a regular journaling process, covering some or all of the following points.

● Journaling requires commitment—at least 30 minutes a week, at a regular time, to be alone and explore feelings by writing and reading.

● Although profound insights may not occur at every session, journaling often prevents us from being the victims of our own biographies.

● This technique for focusing inward, relaxing and allowing phrases, images and memories to arise spontaneously usually leads to in-depth thinking about life and taking a more active part in shaping it.

VARIATIONS

■ **Conflicts Journal**. Review life conflicts or communication breakdowns and explore alternatives for handling each.

■ **Wellness Journey**. Explore paths taken toward well-being and utilize this writing process to support making positive life changes.

■ **Anger Letter**. Write a journal letter to the person/situation that hurts you, describing the pain in great detail. Spare no adjectives. Do not send the letter but read it at a later time as if you were the recipient and respond back to yourself in writing from that perspective.

■ **Kid Talk**. Record special phrases that your children/loved ones share with you. Reflect back on the meaning and value of these relationships and what you do to preserve them.

■ **Stress Map**. Journal sources of stress and identify alternate coping strategies. Reread the journal in order to map your progress and renew your commitment to goals.

■ **Work Fantasies**. Explore images regarding resolution of on-the-job problems. Journal for frustration relief and enhanced creative problem solving.

■ **Spiritual Process**. For renewed zest and spiritual fulfillment, dialogue in writing the intimate aspects of your spirituality.

■ **Communication Log**. Journal with the intent of sharing what you write with a loved one. Reflections of how you are feeling may enhance mutual perceptions and lead to relationship growth and enriched love.

Submitted by David Johnson and Ronda J Salge. Based on concepts from Ira Progoff's **At a Journal Workshop** *(New York: Dialogue House Library, 1981) and Christina Baldwin's* **One on One** *(New York: M Evans and Co, 1977).*

GUIDELINES FOR SELECTING MUSIC

The reason for combining music with the journaling process is to stimulate the limbic system (the feeling part of the brain) so that chemicals will be released in the bloodstream which cause the physiological responses which the brain perceives as emotion.

A key consideration in choice of music is familiarity. If a piece is of an unfamiliar style, participants' expectations will be low and the perceptions experienced during journaling are likely to be less meaningful. Since our expectations are dependent on past experience, we need to provide familiar music that hooks people in right away.

There are pros and cons to both classical and popular pieces. Group participants most often prefer popular songs. Although lyrics may structure associations and projections too much, they are also easily remembered. If a popular song is associated with a new insight through journaling, the song can become a powerful cue for self-help to resolve similar situations in the future. If a specific emotion is targeted for the session, classical pieces may be helpful in eliciting the desired response.

Before choosing music for your session, consider these issues:

* *Is the piece stimulating or sedative?*

* *If your session goal is general self-reflection, are the lyrics reflective and open for interpretation?*

* *If your journaling is aimed toward a specific emotion, is the emotional quality strongly suggested by the music?*

* *If a free flow format is used, you may want a piece that is emotionally ambiguous.*

* *What are the participants' preferences?*

* *Avoid extremes. Experience/experiment with various pieces yourself.*

* *Be cautious of using pieces with which you personally identify strongly.*

91 OPENNESS AND INTIMACY

In this experiment with openness, participants assess their self-disclosure patterns and practice the art of personal sharing.

GOALS

To encourage self-disclosure in personal relationships.

To assess personal styles and patterns of openness.

To practice the art of sharing oneself with others.

GROUP SIZE

Works best with 10–40 participants. With more than 40 people the logistics of the Fishbowl exercise become cumbersome.

TIME FRAME

50–60 minutes

MATERIALS NEEDED

One copy of the **Self-Disclosure and Intimacy** worksheet for each participant.

PHYSICAL SETTING

Movable chairs and plenty of space for several small groups to spread out for the *Fishbowls.*

PROCESS

1) The trainer introduces the exercise with a brief chalktalk on the healthy benefits of openness and intimacy in relationships.

   ● In the 1960's, Sidney Jourard hypothesized that those people who revealed themselves to others would not only live vital, high energy lives, but would also be sick less and would live longer.

   ● This idea was recently substantiated in a landmark health study of 200 men. Over a 40-year period one major factor distinguished those men who were healthy at the end of this time from those who were disabled or had already died: The healthy group reported the consistent presence in their lives of at least one individual with whom they could share their deepest thoughts and feelings.

©1994 Whole Person Press 210 W Michigan Duluth MN 55802   (800) 247-6789

- **Relationships flourish when feelings are shared and understood.** We must be willing to share our feelings if we want others to understand them. When we try to hide our feelings from others we distance ourselves from them and we lose the closeness and support that could comfort and energize us.

- **Sharing ourselves with others is a matter of choice not chance.** Some people choose to be open; others decide to hide their inner self. Many times each day we face the question, "Shall I share myself as I really am, or maintain a 'public self' that camouflages my real self?" Our answers to this question over the days, weeks, and years determine the quality of openness and intimacy we experience in our relationships.

2) The trainer distributes the **Self-Disclosure and Intimacy** worksheets and invites participants to respond in writing to the questions. (5 minutes)

   Before moving to the next step, the trainer asks participants to look over their responses and to make a few mental observations about what they have written and what it may mean to them.

3) Participants are instructed to pair up with a partner and share a few of their observations with each other. (3–4 minutes)

4) The trainer instructs each dyad to gather with 5 other pairs, thus forming a group of 12 people for the exercise to follow, which is called a *Fishbowl.*

   ☞ *You may have to direct this process of group formation. Also, you may alter the number of dyads in a group—depending on the total number of participants. Do not, however, form groups smaller than 5 pairs or larger than 9 pairs.*

   The trainer asks the youngest partner in each pair to gather with the other youngest partners in their group to form an inner circle (seated in chairs). The "leftover" oldest partners in each dyad form an outer ring standing around the seated circle in the middle.

5) The trainer gives instructions to the *outer circle* (*observers*) first.

   ➤ The inner circle will be holding a discussion.

   ➤ During this discussion you are to observe your partner. Be aware of what your partner discloses about herself both by words and by non-verbal behaviors. Check out whether your partner participates as you would expect, based on your knowledge of her **Self-Disclosure and Intimacy** worksheet observations.

➤ Please feel free to move around the circle to a position where you can best hear and see your partner.

6) The trainer then gives directions to the *inner circle.*

➤ You are to hold a 10 minute group meeting on the following questions:

➤ "How do I personally try to cover up my feelings through voice, actions and words . . . and in what situations am I most likely to cover them up?"

➤ Every group member should contribute to the discussion.

7) The trainer checks to make sure everyone understands the process and then signals for the *Fishbowl* exercise to begin.

8) After 10 minutes, the trainer interrupts the *Fishbowl* groups and asks participants to return to their original partners for a five-minute debriefing of the *Fishbowl* experience.

The trainer describes the format for sharing:

➤ The younger shares first, telling how she felt during the *Fishbowl* discussion and reflecting on her process of self-disclosure.

➤ Then the observer tells his partner what he noticed about her verbal and non-verbal self-disclosure.

➤ You will have about 5 minutes. Be sure both people get air time!

☞ *This interchange is not to be judgmental or confrontive! Merely reflective. Be sure the partners listen to each other!*

9) The trainer reforms the *Fishbowl* groups with the second partner now in the inside group. The trainer repeats the instructions for the *observers* (*Step 5*), then instructs the inner circle as follows:

➤ You are to hold a 10-minute group meeting on the following question:

➤ "What feelings do I have trouble expressing and sharing with others . . . and in what situations is this most difficult for me?"

➤ Every group member should contribute to the discussion!

10) As before (*Step 8*), after 10 minutes the trainer interrupts the *Fishbowl* groups and allows partners time to reflect with each other. The partner

who has just been in the *Fishbowl* shares his reactions first. Then the *observer* shares. (5 minutes)

☞ *Remind participants again that listening and acceptance are the foci, not confrontation or judgment.*

11) The trainer reconvenes the entire group and solicits observations from the group, both on the process of this exercise and on the patterns of openness and selfdisclosure evidenced by the group during the exercise.

12) Participants are asked to consider one concluding challenge. The trainer asks everyone to identify a feeling, issue or experience they have never before shared with anyone, that they would be willing to disclose to someone during the next week.

Participants are instructed to identify by name the *person* with whom they will share this secret and set a *date* by when they will do so.

☞ *You might caution the group about what they choose to disclose, saying something like, "Don't share anything that will hurt the other person. What you share must do no harm to others . . . or it won't be healing for you!"*

TRAINER'S NOTES

SELF-DISCLOSURE AND INTIMACY

The quality of your relationships and your intimacy with others is directly related to how much of yourself you're willing to share with them, as well as the degree of support and care you feel for them.

Which of the following are true of your experiences in relationships at this moment?

I have someone in my life with whom I would talk about anything and everything.	Y N
I keep in close touch with my extended family.	Y N
When I need help or emotional support I ask for it directly.	Y N
I meet new people easily and enjoy it.	Y N
I often compliment others.	Y N
I find it possible to share whatever I'm feeling with others right when I'm feeling it.	Y N

How fulfilling have your relationships with others been this past week?

Interpersonal relationships are a sure-fire source of renewed energy and vitality if—and only if—you let others know you as you really are so that they can accept and care about the real you!

How many people know you?

_____ 95%-100%   (They know almost everything about me.)
_____ 75%-95%   (I would share almost anything with them if the "time were right.")
_____ 50%-75%   (I would share much, but I also "cover myself" in many ways.)

Of these, who would you say knows you deeply? And understands who you really are now? Who would accept you no matter what? (Name as many as you honestly can. One is essential, three or four are better for you!)

©1994 Whole Person Press 210 W Michigan Duluth MN 55802   (800) 247-6789

In different relationships we decide the balance between "public" and "private" self quite differently. No one should share themselves equally with everyone. But if you share yourself with no one, your overall health is likely to suffer.

What are you willing to share   What are you **not** willing to share
("public self") with your . . .   ("private self")?

Spouse _____   _____

Children_____   _____

Parents _____   _____

Best friend _____   _____

Work associates _____   _____

People in general _____   _____

To what degree is your "public self" different from your "private self?"

What kinds of things have you never shared with anyone? (You may put these down in code.)

How does your self-disclosure differ with men and with women? Why?

©1994 Whole Person Press 210 W Michigan Duluth MN 55802   (800) 247-6789

92 THAT'S THE SPIRIT!

Participants use a simple checklist to assess their current spiritual self-care habits and then review a menu of spirit-related energizers for enhancing health.

GOALS

To assess participants' spiritual life patterns.

To explore spiritual activities that enrich and rituals that refresh.

GROUP SIZE

Unlimited.

TIME FRAME

10–15 minutes

MATERIALS NEEDED

One copy of the **Spiritual Checkup** checklist for each participant.

PROCESS

1) The trainer introduces the concept that attention to the spirit is healthy, backing up this claim with examples such as the following:

- A hospital chaplain studied the outlook of patients who were suffering serious illnesses and facing stressful surgery. He found that those who did not survive the trauma were more likely to have expressed anger, hate, envy and helplessness, while those who did survive were more likely to have expressed "spiritual values" such as love, gratitude, forgiveness and hope.

- Among people studied in Maryland, those who went to church regularly were at "significantly less risk of dying from heart disease than those who went irregularly." (So, go to church—it will do your heart good in more ways than one!)

- Among adults studied in Alameda County, California, the healthiest were people who had good sound connections, a good marriage, church or synagogue membership, and membership in other associations. Many individuals throughout history who have survived incredibly painful ordeals over many years, attribute their survival

©1994 Whole Person Press 210 W Michigan Duluth MN 55802   (800) 247-6789

directly to their strong spiritual faith (eg, Victor Frankl, Mother Teresa, Helen Hays etc).

☞ *See if the group can help you name a few more!*

2) The trainer distributes a copy of the **Spiritual Checkup** checklist to each participant. Participants complete the questionnaire, total their points and analyze their own scores based on the system provided.

3) The trainer invites comments from the group on how they feel about the adequacy of their current style of spiritual self-nourishment.

4) The trainer asks participants for additional examples of spiritual activities that could enrich well-being and rituals that might refresh the spirit.

In closing, the trainer uses the list below to supplement or summarize the group's suggestions.

● **Seek purpose and meaning in life.** Look for opportunities to engage the depth dimension. Discuss values and ethical issues with family, friends, co-workers. Pursue truth. Nurture your faith.

● **Take time for centering.** Open yourself to the message of the Spirit. Study the Bible or other inspirational/devotional materials. Meditate. Pray. Give thanks. Find time for solitude and silence every day.

● **Make worship or other spiritual rituals a top priority.** Prepare with quiet reflection. Participate with enthusiasm. Celebrate.

● **Activate your sense of wonder.** Listen to inspiring music. Explore nature—even in the city. Use all your senses to notice the miracles of creation all around you. Take time off to enjoy aesthetic pleasures.

● **Cultivate an attitude of compassion and giving.** Reach out and let your love flow in small and big ways. Be courteous. Listen. Forgive. Respond to the needs you see. Make a financial and/or time commitment to a worthy cause. Help someone in pain or difficulty. Look for opportunities to act out justice.

*Submitted by Keith Sehnert. The **Spiritual Checkup** is adapted from his book, **The Family Doctor's Health Tips** (Minneapolis: Meadowbrook 1981).*

©1994 Whole Person Press 210 W Michigan Duluth MN 55802   (800) 247-6789

TRAINER'S NOTES

SPIRITUAL CHECKUP

How's your spiritual life?

When was the last time you...
(check the time frame that applies)

	Yesterday/Today	Last Week	Last Month	Last Year	I Don't Remember
1) Shared ten minutes with a child and talked about a common interest?					
2) Went to a regular church, synagogue or religious service?					
3) Helped someone who is less fortunate (in your opinion) than you?					
4) Took a walk in the park or woods with someone you love?					
5) Prayed for someone?					
6) Watched the sun come up (or go down) while at a lake, in the mountains, in the woods, at home or wherever you might be?					
7) Went to a special church, synagogue or religious service (or served on church committees, programs or related service)?					
8) Read the Bible or other inspirational or devotional materials?					
9) Spent fifteen to thirty minutes or more meditating, praying, pondering or reflecting on your purpose in life?					
10) Attended an art exhibition, a theatre or dance performance or a concert featuring religious works? Listened to an uplifting radio program or recorded music?					
A) Score per check	6	4	2	1	0
B) # of checks in column					
C) Column score (AxB)					

TOTAL SCORE _____

ANALYSIS

After computing your total score (the sum of all column scores), use the general guidelines below for interpreting your results.

Score	Interpretation
40-60	You are probably enjoying all the benefits of a spiritually rich life.
30-39	You have a good emphasis on spiritual values in your life.
20-29	Spiritual concerns are part of your life, but you may want to spend more time concentrating on them.
0-19	Your spiritual life is underdeveloped. Try to bring these values into the limelight, even if it takes some extra effort on your part.

©1994 Whole Person Press 210 W Michigan Duluth MN 55802   (800) 247-6789

93 FOOTLOOSE AND FANCY FREE

This fantasy invites participants to visualize a course for their lives unencumbered by possessions, responsibilities and commitments.

GOALS

To illustrate the fact that the pursuit of material possessions and professional success as ends in themselves may entrap one in unrewarding patterns of living.

To help participants clarify the values and goals that are of deepest importance to them.

To help participants visualize specific lifestyle adjustments they may wish to make for themselves.

GROUP SIZE

Unlimited.

TIME FRAME

10–20 minutes

PROCESS

1) The trainer may open the exercise with a chalktalk outlining the following points and asking participants to reflect on the questions that follow each statement.

  ● The pursuit of possessions for their own sake (and money for its own sake) tend to complicate and clutter one's life—clouding your deeper purpose. Thoreau once said, "It's not the $100 one pays for something that is significant, but the amount of time one spends doing what he does not really want to in order to get that $100. Each luxury adds up and eventually one spends more time earning a living than living."

   ➤ How much of your *living* do you "waste" to gain money for luxuries you don't need?

  ● While a profitable bottom line may be the purpose of a business, it is not an appropriate purpose-of-life for the person in business. Having enough to satisfy one's needs is important. But how much is enough?

➤ What pressures do you experience in keeping up the financial commitments of a lifestyle built on "more than enough?"

● Persons of unusual clarity often voluntarily live a life of simplicity. This simplicity does not necessarily mean "having less" or "returning to a primitive rural life." Rather, it is an attitude which, when adopted, unburdens one from the self-imposed clutter and distraction that get in the way of living.

➤ In what ways is your life unnecessarily complicated?

2) The trainer asks participants to sit back and relax, close their eyes and imagine that they are on a trip. After all have quieted, the trainer reads the **Footloose and Fancy Free Fantasy script,** allowing ample time for participants to visualize each scene and to register their reactions to each question.

☞ *You may need to repeat the last paragraph once or twice, until all have begun writing, but don't break the mood!*

3) The trainer divides participants into groups of three persons each (or pairs if time is short) and asks them to share the details of their "trip." Participants are to focus on the aspects of their current life they were most ready to leave behind and the resolutions for change that these insights suggest.

4) After the trainer reconvenes the entire group, he may point out that effective planning for wellness begins with a reclarifying of life's essentials—as based on one's individual values and beliefs.

VARIATION

■ This self-care consciousness raiser may be used alone, or combined with a specific step-by-step goal setting process.

FOOTLOOSE AND FANCY FREE FANTASY Script

Imagine that you are in a car. You are driving out of town, away from your home.

    ☞ *(Pause 20 seconds)*

Where are you going? Where are you on the journey? Is there anyone with you?

    ☞ *(Pause)*

Imagine that there's no going home. You can never return—never call home—there's no going home.

You own only what you have with you now. You have no responsibilities to return to, no bills, no possessions, no records, no people except those with you—you are free.

    ☞ *(Pause)*

What will you do with your life now
Where will you go?
Who will you see?

    ☞ *(Pause)*

Notice which aspects of your previous life you feel relieved to leave behind . . . and which you will miss.

    ☞ *(Pause)*

What will you do with the rest of this week?
What will you do with the rest of this year
What will you do with the rest of your life?

    ☞ *(Pause)*

Please come back into the room . . . just enough to jot some notes on your images and insights.

    ☞ *(Pause)*

Quietly, by yourself, write some notes about those goals, activities and pressures you felt relieved to leave behind . . . and those you recreated in your new life, because they were so important to you.

    ☞ *(Pause 5 minutes)*

TRAINER'S NOTES

94 POLAROID PERSPECTIVES

In this unusual action metaphor participants compare their personal development to a polaroid snapshot, projecting into the future to imagine how the ever-sharpening outline of their lives will develop.

GOALS

To help participants appreciate the growth and development that they have already experienced.

To stimulate an attitude of self-responsibility.

GROUP SIZE

Any size. Works well with individuals and/or families.

TIME FRAME

30–50 minutes

MATERIALS NEEDED

One Polaroid camera with flash and film; one copy of **My Developing Perspectives** and **My Developing Snapshot** worksheets for each participant.

PROCESS

1) The trainer enters the room and says nothing. She begins by silently taking Polaroid snapshots of the group, or various subgroups. As she snaps pictures of participants she hands the undeveloped photo to them saying:

   ➤ Please sit in silence for two minutes and watch yourself develop. Everything will become clear in its own time . . . just as it always does!

   She then moves on to take a picture of the next subgroup and repeats the process.

2) After all pictures have been taken and the time for development has elapsed, the trainer asks the group to share their reactions, and the ideas that crossed their minds about the meaning of this process. On the blackboard, the trainer lists all the possibilities that are suggested, without commenting.

©1994 Whole Person Press 210 W Michigan Duluth MN 55802   (800) 247-6789

3) The trainer elaborates on the polaroid snapshot as a metaphor for personal development and self-responsibility, illustrating the chalk-talk with insights participants have shared and the concepts outlined below:

- Like an undeveloped Polaroid snapshot, the current events of our lives often look blank, or at best unclear. Through time, situations develop their own outline and our perspective becomes clear.

- We are still developing—not in two minutes, but over our entire lifetime. Our structure becomes clear, our patterns emerge and the intricacies of our unique styles are colored in deeper and richer hues. Our outlines take form slowly over time.

- Just as some snapshots are less clear than others, (being underexposed, double images, out of focus or overexposed), so also some elements in our lives may remain less than perfectly clear even after they are fully developed.

- We have an impact on the kind of picture that emerges from our life. We are always making and remaking decisions—where and how to spend our selves, the commitments we make, our answers to moral dilemmas. With each investment decision we determine our emerging outline—we shape the details of our developing selves.

4) The trainer distributes **My Developing Perspectives** worksheets to participants and asks them to complete the questions on the top third of the page.

☞ *Encourage people to recall the images they experienced as they watched the Polaroid photo of their subgroup develop. They are to make notes of images, vague notions and subtle hints that occur to them about their current developmental issues.*

You may want to give a few examples of your own (eg, "I'm not sure whether I'm in the right job, but over the next six months it will get clearer and clearer," or "I'm on the verge of a whole new friendship and all that it can mean.")

You also may need to remind participants that they are noting issues that are unclear, since by definition they're not yet developed. People will need to rely on their intuition and image system to answer the questions.

5) As soon as most people are finished, the trainer instructs participants to complete the bottom two-thirds of the worksheet, writing their responses to the six questions.

©1994 Whole Person Press 210 W Michigan Duluth MN 55802   (800) 247-6789

6) The trainer distributes one copy of the **My Developing Snapshot** worksheet to each participant. She invites participants to draw an instant Polaroid of their lives at this moment using the images identified in the **My Developing Perspectives** worksheet.

➤ Include in your picture:
  ➤ The broad outlines that have already become focused over the years.
  ➤ The emerging structure of your life.
  ➤ The vague, hazy issues that have yet to appear in recognizable form.

➤ Take three minutes to develop your picture!

7) After three minutes, participants are instructed to stop drawing and take a look at their picture.

➤ Study your picture for one minute, noticing what you have drawn—some details clearly, some out of focus, some only vague notions.

☞ *Pause for one minute.*

➤ Now take another three minutes to sharpen your personal snapshot.
  ➤ Add focus as needed, clarify additional issues and structural elements as seems appropriate.

8) The trainer divides participants into groups of 3–4 persons each, or utilizes previously established discussion/sharing units. She instructs them to show their Polaroid pictures to each other, using the format below.

➤ Take turns. When it is your turn, point out in your picture the elements that depict:
  ➤ Two dimensions of my life that have become very clear over the years.
  ➤ Two issues in my life that are currently emerging, but are not yet fully outlined.
  ➤ Two elements in my life that are still too vague to label, but I know they are present and that they will emerge in future years.

☞ *List these past, present, future questions on the blackboard or newsprint for easy reference.*

➤ Each person should take about 5 minutes to show your Polaroid snapshot and elaborate on the details.

9) The trainer reconvenes the group and closes the exercise by receiving whatever final observations and comments the group wishes to offer.

VARIATIONS

■ If the participants have already been divided into discussion/sharing subgroups prior to this session, the trainer may wish to have them gather into these groups at the beginning of the session. Then the trainer could take a Polaroid photo of each discussion group.

■ Later, following the session, the actual Polaroid photo and the **My Developing Snapshot** self portraits for the members of each group could be posted on the walls around the room.

■ If the training event entails multiple sessions, the trainer may ask participants to bring their **My Developing Snapshots** to later sessions and instruct participants then to draw more clearly the details that have emerged during the time that has elapsed between sessions.

The inspiration for this exercise came from a children's sermon delivered by Rev Liz Oettinger, Portland OR.

MY DEVELOPING PERSPECTIVES

What issues/events in your life currently look and feel confusing? Undeveloped? Unclear? **Confusing Issue/event:**	How do you imagine each one will develop during the next 3 months, 6 months or a year? **My hunch is this will . . .**

The outlines that have developed already . . .

List one aspect of your life that is clear today, but was not clear last week.

List one issue in your life that is clear today, but was not clear last week.

List one major dimension of your life that is clear today, but was not clear five years ago.

The outlines to come . . .

List one aspect of your life that is unclear today, but should be clear by next week.

List one issue in your life that is unclear today, but will probably be developed by next year at this time.

List one major dimension of your life that is vague today, but will probably have taken shape five years from now.

©1994 Whole Person Press 210 W Michigan Duluth MN 55802   (800) 247-6789

MY DEVELOPING SNAPSHOT

©1994 Whole Person Press 210 W Michigan Duluth MN 55802   (800) 247-6789

TRAINER'S NOTES

Planning
& Closure

95 CLOSING STATEMENTS

In this reflective and integrative process participants pull together insights from the learning experience and assess its impact on them.

GOALS

To provide closure for the learning experience.

To reinforce discoveries, insights and resolutions made during the session.

GROUP SIZE

Unlimited.

TIME FRAME

10–30 minutes

MATERIALS NEEDED

Closing Statements worksheets for all participants.

PROCESS

1) The trainer announces that the remainder of the session will be devoted to personal reflection, application and assessment of the learning experience. He distributes **Closing Statements** worksheets to participants and invites them to respond in writing to each statement.

   ☞ *Encourage people to answer thoughtfully and in as much detail as they choose. They may need a reminder not to get bogged down—it's okay to leave some items blank if nothing comes to mind.*

2) After about 10 minutes, the trainer invites participants to choose one of their completed statements to read to the group.

   ☞ *Be sure to write and share your own closing statements.*

3) If time remains after everyone has had a turn, the trainer may open the floor to further sharing of closing statements before dismissing the group.

VARIATION

■ To add a little spice to the sharing process, participants could pair up with a series of partners, sharing a different response with each person. *Two Minute Mill* (**Wellness 1,** p 5) and *Closing Formation* (**Stress 3,** p 97) describe unusual techniques for pairing and sharing.

TRAINER'S NOTES

CLOSING STATEMENTS

Complete each of the statements below with a phrase that applies to your participation in this learning experience.

1) I learned that . . .

2) I rediscovered that . . .

3) I changed my mind about . . .

4) I realized that I . . .

5) I had the most difficulty with . . .

6) The high point for me was . . .

7) I especially want to remember . . .

8) I certainly appreciated . . .

9) I am looking forward to . . .

10) I am determined to . . .

11) As a result of this experience I . . .

©1994 Whole Person Press 210 W Michigan Duluth MN 55802   (800) 247-6789

96 DAILY WELLNESS GRAPH

Participants learn how to chart the daily ups and downs of their progress toward higher levels of wellness.

GOALS

To heighten awareness of the change process.

To provide feedback about wellness-oriented behaviors in several life dimensions.

GROUP SIZE

Works best with a smaller group of participants who are committed to behavior change; also works well one-to-one.

TIME FRAME

20–30 minutes for introduction; 5 minutes daily for a month.

MATERIALS NEEDED

Wellness Lifestyle Dimensions and **Daily Wellness Graph** worksheets for all participants.

PROCESS

1) The trainer begins by asking participants for examples of changes they would like to make, based on what they have learned in the course so far and their desire to pursue a healthier lifestyle.

   If the issues do not come up spontaneously, she asks about potential changes in the areas of *moods and feelings, rest and sleep, nutrition, physical activity, relationships and the environment.* All suggestions are listed on the board.

2) The trainer provides some general information on the nature of the change process as it relates to altering health habits:

   - We human beings are rather resistant to change—change implies adjustment, discomfort and effort. Making lifestyle changes is particularly troublesome since our bad habits usually have enjoyable benefits that are difficult to replace.
   - It typically takes about *two years* for a person to develop a new lifestyle, incorporating a wide spectrum of changes.

©1994 Whole Person Press 210 W Michigan Duluth MN 55802   (800) 247-6789

- It takes about *six months* of practice before a new behavior is integrated enough into one's daily life to feel "natural."
- It takes about *28 days* of repetition to "get the hang of" a specific new behavior.
- Most people need frequent reinforcement in order to initiate and maintain changes.

3) The trainer distributes **Wellness Lifestyle Dimensions** to all and asks participants to jot down, on the left side of the page, several criteria they might use to measure their well-being in each of the lifestyle dimensions (3–5 minutes).

   ☞ *There are no right answers—let people struggle a little and make up their own standards without examples or consultation.*

4) The trainer asks for examples of criteria for each dimension and encourages participants to add to their own list any ideas generated by the group that seem appropriate to them.

5) Participants are instructed to personalize a nine-point self-rating scale on the right hand side of the **Wellness Lifestyle Dimensions** worksheet.

   ➤ In the space below the number scale in each box, list a few signals (behavior, attitude, etc) for each dimension that would mean you are at the *low end* of the scale (1, 2, 3);

   ➤ Then list a few indicators that would signify that you are on the *high end* of the scale (7, 8, 9).

      ☞ *Give some examples for refernece: eg, on the "Mood and Feelings" dimension, the low end might be characterized by depression, feeling guilty or being irritable, while the high end of the scale might be characterized by an upbeat feeling, lots of good laughter and a feeling of competency, etc.*

      You may want to give a few examples of what might push a person's score up and down, but remind people that everyone's standards will be different.

6) After about 5 minutes the trainer distributes **Daily Wellness Graphs** to everyone and explains how to keep track on a daily basis.

   ➤ Since wellness goals and criteria differ from individual to individual, everyone will need to use his or her own nine-point, low to high rating scale.

   ➤ Give yourself wellness scores for *today* and record your scores on the graph.

©1994 Whole Person Press 210 W Michigan Duluth MN 55802   (800) 247-6789

7) The trainer closes the exercise by challenging participants to try the **Wellness Graph** for a week (or month, or until the next class) and offering a few helpful hints. Some or all of the following points could be included.

- This system will not be everyone's cup of tea. Some personality types love numbers and checklists—others abhor them. If you like daily reinforcement, the graph will probably work for you. If not, why not try it anyway. If you're sick and tired of being sick and tired, anything is worth a try!

- Even if you're not trying to change anything, keeping a chart like this for a month will provide a rich source of feedback about your current lifestyle.

- If you are making changes, you will find that this graph takes on the character of a mini-biorhythm chart. As you make changes in one lifestyle dimension, that change will feed positively into other areas creating a domino effect. As a result, you will probably start seeing improvements in other dimensions as well.

- Try to log your scores at the same time every day. Post your graph on the refrigerator or "check-in" with a buddy at work each day. Do pay attention as well to the subtle shifts in attitude and behavior that you experience during the day, and make note of any patterns that you observe.

  ☞ *At the next meeting be sure to set aside time for participants to report on their experience with graphing. For added impact institute a buddy system for check-in and between-session reinforcement.*

Submitted by Jean Mershon who learned a similar process from Ted Tsmura, Denver CO.

WELLNESS LIFESTYLE DIMENSIONS

	LOW							HIGH	
MOOD & FEELINGS	1	2	3	4	5	6	7	8	9
REST & SLEEP	1	2	3	4	5	6	7	8	9
NUTRITION	1	2	3	4	5	6	7	8	9
PHYSICAL ACTIVITY	1	2	3	4	5	6	7	8	9
RELATIONAL	1	2	3	4	5	6	7	8	9
ENVIRONMENTAL	1	2	3	4	5	6	7	8	9

©1994 Whole Person Press 210 W Michigan Duluth MN 55802   (800) 247-6789

DAILY WELLNESS GRAPH

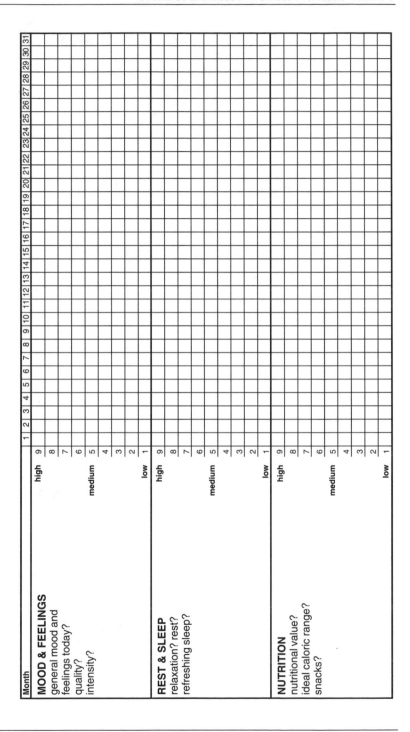

©1994 Whole Person Press 210 W Michigan Duluth MN 55802 (800) 247-6789

DAILY WELLNESS GRAPH, part 2

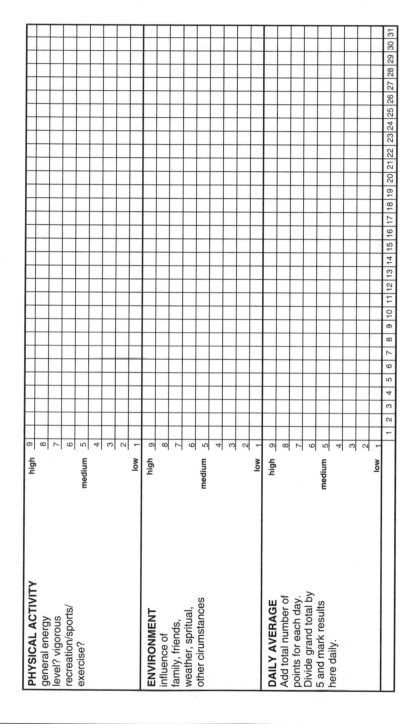

PHYSICAL ACTIVITY
general energy
level? vigorous
recreation/sports/
exercise?

ENVIRONMENT
influence of
family, friends,
weather, spritual,
other cirumstances

DAILY AVERAGE
Add total number of
points for each day.
Divide grand total by
5 and mark results
here daily.

©1994 Whole Person Press 210 W Michigan Duluth MN 55802   (800) 247-6789

97 FORTUNE COOKIES

Participants invent wellness fortunes for one another and exchange them in unusual "cookies."

GOALS

To reinforce wellness concepts.

To articulate desired goals and changes.

To provide an upbeat closing to the session.

GROUP SIZE

Unlimited, but more time-consuming and chaotic with a larger group.

TIME FRAME

15–20 minutes

MATERIALS NEEDED

Balloons and small strips of paper for each person; the exercise is more fun when participants have two or more balloons. Blackboard or newsprint.

PROCESS

1) The trainer invites participants to review the issues and concerns raised during the session/course/workshop, remembering specific **concepts** they want to apply, wellness **behaviors** they want to incorporate into their lifestyle, wellness **goals** they hope to attain, **ideas** for further exploration, **discoveries** they have made about wellness, etc.

   She solicits examples of wellness goals, plans for behavior change and other desired applications of the course content. Each insight and idea for implementation is recorded on the blackboard or on several sheets of newsprint displayed across the front of the room.

2) After a multitude of ideas have been generated, the trainer announces that participants will now have an unusual opportunity to support each other's wellness goals by writing messages of encouragement in the form of the proverbial fortune cookie.

   The trainer distributes balloons and strips of paper to everyone. She describes the process and parameters of writing fortunes, giving several appropriate examples at each step.

> Choose a wellness concept, goal or application from the list generated by the group (eg, lose weight, pay attention to spiritual growth, being responsible for my own well-being, etc).

> Make up a fortune that predicts *successful* attainment of the goal or implementation of the concept (eg, "You will reach and maintain your ideal weight"). Add a touch of humor, if possible (eg, "You will lose your taste for chocolate chip cookies and receive a thousand compliments on your vanishing cellulite this year").

Your fortune could also take the form of an aphorism, motto or other words of wisdom (eg, "Cultivate the attitude of gratitude"). Again, creativity and humor will make the fortune more memorable (eg, "Dance for the health of it!").

> All fortunes should be positive and affirming. No sarcasm, cynicism or put-downs allowed!

> Write one fortune on each slip of paper. Then blow up the balloon (with the fortune inside) and tie it.

3) Participants are instructed to exchange fortune cookies by batting their balloons in the air, keeping all balloons off the ground for one minute.

After one minute, the trainer interrupts the chaos and directs participants to capture as many balloons as they originally launched, being careful not to break them.

4) The trainer asks participants to notice the color of the first balloon they captured. She designates different areas of the room for each color and directs participants to move to the area that matches their first choice balloon color.

After people have gathered into groups by color, the trainer announces that these small groups will have about 10 minutes to tell their fortunes.

> Take turns "opening" your fortune "cookies," reading the messages out loud and sharing with each other any personal resolutions for change you have made as a result of this learning experience.

5) The trainer reconvenes the total group and asks for examples of exceptionally clever or meaningful fortunes.

After several people have shared, she closes the meeting by reading a fortune cookie message she has written especially for the group that predicts for them a successful increase in their positive health behaviors.

VARIATION

■ With 20 people or less, there is no need to divide into groups for *Step 4.*

TRAINER'S NOTES

©1994 Whole Person Press 210 W Michigan Duluth MN 55802   (800) 247-6789

98 HEALTH REPORT CARD

In this closing ritual, small groups of participants affirm one another's positive health habits.

GOALS

To provide closure to the group experience.

To reinforce positive health habits and attitudes.

GROUP SIZE

Unlimited.

TIME FRAME

25–30 minutes with 4-person sharing groups; more with larger groups.

MATERIALS NEEDED

Enough 3x5 cards so that each participant has one for each member of her group.

PROCESS

☞ *This exercise is most effective with groups where people know each other well or where small sharing groups have met several times during an extended learning experience.*

1) The trainer instructs participants to rejoin their small groups (or form new groups of four) and find a comfortable place in the room.

   As soon as everyone has found a spot, the trainer distributes a stack of 3x5 cards to each group and announces that during the next half hour participants will have an opportunity to evaluate the benefits of this course by affirming wellness-oriented behaviors they have observed in themselves and others.

2) The trainer directs the groups through the first part of the process.

   ➤ Pass the index cards around your group. Each person should take enough so that you have a different card for every person in the group, including yourself.

   ➤ On each card, write the name of a different group member. Don't forget yourself.

➤ These cards represent "report cards" on which you will be giving positive feedback about each person's wellness lifestyle. When you think about each person's wellness lifestyle, consider habits, behaviors, attitudes, values, etc, that you have noticed.

➤ Write a "report card" for each person in your group. Think about the qualities of vitality and well-being you have observed in that person.

    ➣ List on the card three positive health habits or attributes you admire in that person (eg, daily exercise, cat naps, faith guides life, optimistic attitude, stops eating when full, etc).

    ➣ Don't forget the whole person perspective—body, mind, spirit, and interpersonal well-being are all worthy of commendation.

    ➣ Be specific and personal—make each card unique! Be sure to fill out a report card for yourself, too.

➤ Sign each report card.

    ☞ *Adjust the timing here to match the size of the group. People will probably need about 2 minutes for each report card. If some people finish early, encourage them to go back and add some details to their affirmations. Give people a few minutes warning so they can finish up before you move on to the next step.*

3) The trainer regains the attention of the group, explains how they are to conduct the feedback process and clarifies any questions that arise.

➤ The person whose first name comes first in the alphabet begins.

    ➣ Go around the group telling each person directly the qualities you appreciate, giving specific examples of when you observed the value, attitude or behavior in action.

    ➣ Then hand the person his report card. It should take about 3–4 minutes for one person to hand out all your report cards.

    ➣ Save your own report card for the next step.

➤ After each person has given and received appreciation from every group member, it is time for self-affirmation.

    ➣ Each person in turn read your own self-report card out loud and comment briefly on how this learning experience has positively impacted on your well-being (2 minutes each).

4) The trainer gives the signal for groups to begin the sharing process and periodically announces the time remaining so that groups can pace their sharing. (20 minutes)

©1994 Whole Person Press 210 W Michigan Duluth MN 55802   (800) 247-6789

5) The trainer reconvenes the large group and asks participants to give him a report card. Participants are invited to describe what they have appreciated about the learning experience—sharing examples of content or process that have been particularly meaningful.

TRAINER'S NOTES

TRAINER'S NOTES

©1994 Whole Person Press 210 W Michigan Duluth MN 55802   (800) 247-6789

Group
Energizers

99 50 EXCUSES FOR A CLOSED MIND

This humorous list exposes the resistance to new ideas for what it is—rationalization for keeping a closed mind.

GOALS

To illustrate how excuses deaden creativity.

To discover personal styles of resisting the new.

GROUP SIZE

Unlimited.

TIME FRAME

5–15 minutes

MATERIALS NEEDED

Small slips of paper, each with a separate **Excuse for a Closed Mind**—to be prepared ahead of time.

☞ *Don't be limited by the 50 phrases as you prepare the "written excuses." Pick and choose those that fit your audience. Your own creative additions will make the exercise more enjoyable and relevant to the group.*

PROCESS

1) The trainer distributes slips of paper, each containing a different **Excuse for a Closed Mind.**

   Participants who receive an "excuse slip" are instructed to hold it until the trainer says, ***"What do you think?"*** When participants hear that phrase they are one-by-one to express their excuses loudly and clearly.

2) The trainer presents a brief chalktalk on the relationship between creativity and open-mindedness.

   ● The human mind is an incredible source of vitality. Every new idea that we entertain leaves a sparkle of energy.

   ● Unfortunately, most people close their minds—at least in certain situations or about specific issues. Rather than risk the upheavel of new approaches—even though they might be revitalizing—we

©1994 Whole Person Press 210 W Michigan Duluth MN 55802   (800) 247-6789

instead defend the comfortable and familiar using a host of excuses that drive away new ideas before they can ever be taken seriously.

● What a shame! Eventually this shutting down process will virtually guarantee boring and dull lives—when nothing new gets through.

● In this exercise, we will experiment with the energy-depleting power of excuses that protect us from new ideas and keep our minds closed.

3) The trainer closes the chalktalk with the following question:

✔ I'd like you to help me with this experiment. It should be quite different and stimulating! *What do you think?*

☞ *This is the signal for audience participation. If necessary, prompt participants to take turns shouting out the excuses listed in their papers. From time to time you can pick up the pace by reiterating your challenge, "I'd like you to help me with this experiment. It should be fun.* **What do you think?***"*

4) The trainer and participants go back and forth in this manner as the tempo and volume rises, until all the excuses have been expressed.

5) The trainer leads a discussion of the reactions and feelings generated by this exercise.

☞ *Be sure to share what happened to your energy as the group repeatedly resisted your efforts.*

VARIATIONS

■ The written excuses could be personalized by the trainer to fit the specific needs, jargon or character of the group. For a student group include a few excuses like, "Fine—but will it help me write my paper?" or "How gross!" For a business group, "This won't improve the bottom line."

■ The group may be invited to add to the list of excuses, or to make up an entire list of their own.

■ At the beginning of the exercise, the trainer may ask two or three people to stand up front to soak up the impact of all the excuses. At the conclusion of the exercise these participants are interviewed about how it felt to get so totally "shot down."

Submitted by Joel Goodman.

©1994 Whole Person Press 210 W Michigan Duluth MN 55802   (800) 247-6789

50 EXCUSES FOR A CLOSED MIND

1) You've gone too far!

2) We did all right without it.

3) It's never been tried before.

4) I know a person who tried it.

5) It won't work in our plant/office.

6) That's too ivory tower.

7) It's too much trouble to change.

8) Let's shelve it for the time being.

9) We've always done it this way.

10) We'd lose money in the long run.

11) Watch yourself, buddy!

12) Has anyone else ever tried it?

13) Where'd you dig that one up?

14) Good thought, but impractical.

15) Can't teach an old dog new tricks.

16) Let's look into it further.

17) The staff will never buy it.

18) It's against company policy.

19) We don't have the authority.

20) We'll be the laughing stock.

21) Top management won't buy it.

22) Let's give it more thought.

23) We tried that before.

24) It costs too much!

25) It's too radical a change.

26) We don't have the time.

27) Our place is different.

28) Let's get back to reality.

29) I don't like that idea.

30) We're not ready for that.

31) It's too much work!

32) Let's form a committee.

33) Let's all sleep on it.

34) It won't pay for itself.

35) Don't rock the boat!

36) Quit dreaming!

37) The union will scream.

38) That's not my job.

39) They're too busy to do that.

40) There's not enough help.

41) Runs up our overhead.

42) That's not our problem.

43) You're right, but . . .

44) It isn't in the budget.

45) Not that again!

46) I don't see the connection.

47) It can't be done.

48) It's impossible!

49) You're two years ahead of your time.

50) The executive committee would never go for it

©1994 Whole Person Press 210 W Michigan Duluth MN 55802   (800) 247-6789

100 BREATHING ELEMENTS

Participants draw strength and relaxation from imaging their connection with the four basic elements: earth, air, fire and water.

GOALS

To focus attention on conscious breathing.

To enhance relaxation by visualizing images of nature and the basic physical elements.

GROUP SIZE

Any size group is appropriate.

TIME FRAME

5 minutes

PROCESS

1) The trainer instructs participants to relax comfortably in a chair with eyes closed, spine straight, feet flat on the floor and palms face up in their laps.

2) The trainer guides participants through the four breathing patterns using the images and sequence outlined in the **Breathing Elements** script.

   ☞ *Be sure to allow time for participants to quiet and get settled before beginning. Then read the script slowly, in a relaxed voice, allowing ample transition time between each separate image.*

   Do not rush participants at the conclusion. It may take 30 – 40 seconds for them to reorient and be ready to move on to the next activity.

VARIATION

■ The trainer may help participants warm up to this visualization by showing a few slides of tall trees, near water, in the sunshine, at sunrise or sunset, with an open sky as background. Or, appropriate slides could be interspersed between each of the four visual elements.

Submitted by Martha Belknap.

©1994 Whole Person Press 210 W Michigan Duluth MN 55802   (800) 247-6789

BREATHING ELEMENTS Script

EARTH

Inhale through your nose . . . exhale through your nose . . .
*Focus on **physical** energy . . .*
*Visualize a **tree** . . . with strong roots, and full branches . . .*
As you inhale, draw in strength . . . health . . . security . . . power . . .

As you exhale affirm to yourself:
> *I draw strength from the earth . . .*
> *I am grounded like a tree.*

WATER

Inhale through your nose . . . exhale through your mouth . . .
*Focus on **mental** energy . . .*
Visualize a flowing stream . . . with clear, cool water . . .
As you inhale, draw in freedom . . . clarity . . . spontaneity . . .
As you exhale affirm:
> *I draw freedom from the water . . .*
> *I am flowing like a stream.*

FIRE

Inhale through your mouth . . . exhale through your nose . . .
*Focus on **emotional** energy . . .*
Visualize the radiant sunshine . . . with its brightness and heat . . .
As you inhale, draw in warmth . . . light . . . love . . . joy . . .
laughter . . .
As you exhale affirm:
> *I draw warmth from the sun . . .*
> *I am radiant like the sun.*

AIR

Inhale through your mouth . . . exhale through your mouth . . .
*Focus on **spiritual** energy . . .*
Visualize the open air . . . the wind . . . the clouds . . .
As you inhale, draw in awareness . . . expansion . . .
As you exhale affirm:
> *I draw openness from the wind . . .*
> *I am expanding like the air.*

Allow your breathing to return to normal . . .
> *Begin to stretch very slowly . . .*
> *Open your eyes when you are ready . . .*
> *Bring your attention back into the room.*

©1994 Whole Person Press 210 W Michigan Duluth MN 55802   (800) 247-6789

101 THE FEELINGS FACTORY

This energy stretch break demonstrates how various physical actions can generate a plethora of different feelings.

GOALS

To energize the group.

To demonstrate the close connection between our physical activities and our feelings.

TIME FRAME

2–3 minutes

PROCESS

1) The trainer announces that she is going to lead the group through a sequence of physical activities that are likely to evoke feelings. She invites participants to identify and shout out loud the feelings that they experience as they are doing each activity.

   ☞ *Demonstrate one or two actions, shouting out the associated feelings and prodding participants to do the same until everyone gets the idea.*

   Point out that people may experience different—or changing— feelings in response to the same movement. Encourage people to articulate their changing feelings.

2) The trainer selects about a dozen activity options from the **Feelings Factory Actions** list and leads the group through the series, announcing a new activity every 10–15 seconds. Participants shout out the feelings they experience as they act out the movements.

   ☞ *Be sure to encourage participants to keep shouting out the feelings that they experience!*

3) As participants settle back into their chairs, the trainer invites them to briefly share comments on this experience.

©1994 Whole Person Press 210 W Michigan Duluth MN 55802   (800) 247-6789

FEELINGS FACTORY ACTIONS List

* Wave your fists in the air.

* Hold your arms straight out, palms facing forward in a "halt" motion.

* Lock your knees, make your body stiff and rigid.

* Shake your head sideways (as if to say "no").

* Nod your head up and down (as if to say "yes").

* Slump your shoulders, drop your chin and stick out your lower lip.

* Wave (as if "hello" or "good-bye").

* Stamp your feet.

* Clap loudly.

* Throw an elbow (as if to knock something/someone).

* Wave your arm and hand in a "come to me" motion.

* Collapse totally.

* Stretch your arms overhead and relax with a deep breath.

* Rotate your pelvis (or try pelvic thrusts)!

* Scratch your head.

* Shrug your shoulders.

* Smile with your whole face.

* Slap your knee.

* Lift your chin high, with nose up in the air.

* Fold your arms and turn your back.

* Tap your foot rapidly.

* Open your eyes wide.

* Open yourself—extend your arms as if ready for an embrace.

102 LIMERICKS

In small groups, participants compose witty ditties with a wellness theme.

GOALS

To stimulate creativity and humor.

To reinforce wellness concepts.

GROUP SIZE

Unlimited.

TIME FRAME

15–20 minutes

MATERIALS

Limericks worksheets for all participants.

PROCESS

☞ *This process works especially well with small groups who have already spent time sharing and working together.*

1) The trainer reconvenes small groups (or instructs participants to form triads or quartets) and distributes **Limericks** worksheets to all.

2) The trainer announces that participants will be composing group limericks that illustrate wellness concepts of their choice (eg, the nature of dis-ease in our culture, the search for wholeness, the perils of poor self-care habits, the benefits of a wellness lifestyle, etc). The final products can be serious or humorous.

She reviews the meter and rhyme pattern of limericks, as outlined on the worksheet and reads a few sample limericks to set the mood.

☞ *Most people are familiar with limericks, but be prepared with lots of examples to stimulate creativity. Include some humorous—or even spicy—limericks, along with some wellness-oriented ones like this:*

> *If you want to be well in this day,*
> *Eat less fats, hit the trail so they say.*
> *Then challenge your mind,*

©1994 Whole Person Press 210 W Michigan Duluth MN 55802   (800) 247-6789

To your soul be quite kind,
Then healthy and whole you will stay.

Participants are challenged to spend about 10 minutes working together as a group to create one or more limericks.

☞ *Be sure to have one or more rhyming dictionaries available for consultation. You may want to circulate among the groups and offer assistance as needed.*

3) After 10 minutes, the trainer invites each group to read their compositions.

TRAINER'S NOTES

LIMERICKS

FORMAT

Each space represents a syllable.
The first syllable (in parentheses) is used only occasionally, to squeeze in an extra word.
Marked (´) syllables are accented.

Line 1 (___) ___ ___´ ___ ___ ___´ ___ ___ ___´

Line 2 (___) ___ ___´ ___ ___ ___´ ___ ___ ___´

Line 3 (___) ___ ___´ ___ ___ ___´

Line 4 (___) ___ ___´ ___ ___ ___´

Line 5 (___) ___ ___´ ___ ___ ___´ ___ ___ ___´

Lines 1, 2 and 5 rhyme.
Lines 3 and 4 rhyme

(____) ___ ___ ___ ___ ___ ___ ___ ___

(____) ___ ___ ___ ___ ___ ___ ___ ___
(____) ___ ___ ___ ___ ___

(____) ___ ___ ___ ___ ___

(____) ___ ___ ___ ___ ___ ___ ___ ___

(____) ___ ___ ___ ___ ___ ___ ___ ___

(____) ___ ___ ___ ___ ___ ___ ___ ___
(____) ___ ___ ___ ___ ___

(____) ___ ___ ___ ___ ___

(____) ___ ___ ___ ___ ___ ___ ___ ___

103 BALANCING ACT

Participants pair up to demonstrate the dynamic process of maintaining a healthy balance.

GOALS

To experience the give and take required to maintain balance.

To illustrate the concept and process of balance as a health goal.

TIME FRAME

5–10 minutes

PROCESS

1) The trainer asks everyone to find a partner and move to a spot in the room where they are at least arms-length from all other pairs.

2) Partners are instructed to face each other, about three feet apart. The trainer asks participants to reach out, touch palms with each other and lean forward.

3) The trainer uses the analogy of a bicycle to describe the process of balancing that requires repeated shifts in body weight to stay upright over varying speeds and terrain. The trainer notes that health decisions often require the same kind of ongoing adjustment process to keep oneself in balance.

4) The trainer invites partners to experiment with the balance dilemma themselves. First, one partner takes a small step backwards. When the adjustment to that move has been made and the balance between partners has been recovered, the other partner takes a step backwards.

5) *Step 4* is repeated until partners are leaning their weight forward and relying on the weight of each other to balance themselves.

6) The trainer may ask for observations from the group on the "art of balance" and how it applies to self-care decisions.

©1994 Whole Person Press 210 W Michigan Duluth MN 55802   (800) 247-6789

104 OUTRAGEOUS EPISODES

In this energizer participants recall their most outrageous behavior, and relish the playfulness and the risk-taking embodied in their activity.

GOALS

To highlight the role of risk-taking and playfulness in personal vitality.

To raise the group's energy level as they enjoy the recalling and reading of outrageous behaviors.

GROUP SIZE

At least 30 people to ensure anonymity and a high level of creativity—the more the merrier.

TIME FRAME

5–10 minutes

MATERIALS NEEDED

Blank paper.

PROCESS

1) The trainer asks participants to recall the most outrageous thing they ever did. They are to write it down on a blank sheet of paper, but are not to identify themselves on the paper.

   ☞ *You may need to give people a little time to stimulate their thinking with a few examples of your own. Assure them that their contribution will remain anonymous. Joke about this being confession time. Acknowledge that they may have never told anyone about this. Encourage their laughter and smiles as these start to appear around the room. Exhort them to write down* **The Most Outrageous** *behavior!*

2) Participants are asked to stand. The trainer instructs them to crush their sheet of paper into a tight wad. Then, at the count of three they are to throw their paper.

   ➤ "All together now, one . . . two . . . three . . . THROW!"

©1994 Whole Person Press 210 W Michigan Duluth MN 55802   (800) 247-6789

3) Participants are invited to find one crumpled paper near them, then open it up and read it. If they don't like the one they picked up they may crumple it and throw it again—and then go in search of another. When they find one they think is particularly "juicy" they are instructed to bring it up to the trainer.

4) Amidst the confusion, as the trainer receives selected outrageous episodes, he begins reading out loud the best of those he receives— making any additional comments as he sees fit (eg, "Were you arrested?" "Oh, I couldn't possibly read this one out loud," etc).

☞ *You may want to have a few of your own outrageous examples in mind, in case your early receipts are a bit dull (eg, "Mooned my mother while she was meeting with an insurance salesman," "Played softball in a tux," "Lustfully tore the white shirt off my husband at the dinner table while my children watched.").*

If the group is particularly raucous, you may also comment, "Well, I surely had no idea you folks were like this!"

5) After a number of samples have been read, but while the energy in the room is still high, the trainer says "Stop! How do you feel right now?" Participants share comments on how they are feeling at the moment. The trainer encourages participants to hang on to the feelings of energy and well-being that prevail amidst the laughter.

6) In closing, the trainer elicits a discussion on the effect that the willingness to play and the capacity to take risks has on our sense of well-being.

VARIATION

■ The trainer may collect as many outrageous episodes as possible, have them typed, duplicated and distributed to the participants. This written record would serve as a reminder of this exercise, and of the energy that outrageous play can generate.

Submitted by Earl Hipp.

©1994 Whole Person Press 210 W Michigan Duluth MN 55802   (800) 247-6789

105 SAY THE MAGIC WORD

In this short, simple exercise participants design their own vitality formula and capsulize it into a personal "magic word."

GOALS

To identify the personal energizers that frequently brighten one's day.

To devise a unique personal reminder that will help recall these surefire nourishers whenever they are needed.

GROUP SIZE

Unlimited.

TIME REQUIRED

5–10 minutes

MATERIALS NEEDED

Blank paper.

PROCESS

1) The trainer distributes blank paper and gives instructions for creating a "magic word."

   ➤ List five things from your normal environment that are guaranteed to bring a smile to your face and to lighten your hearts.

   These should be people, activities, objects or memories that are readily available to you most of the time. (For example, the smile of a special friend, an enthusiastic pet, a special photo, one's children, a ritual of hugging, a favorite chair, etc.)

   ➤ Next, identify and write down a *one word label* for each of these energizers (eg, smile, Rover, photo, Andy, hugs, etc).

   ➤ Finally, list the first letter of each energizer separately on your paper (eg, S, R, P, A, H). and rearrange these five letters into a word—your personal "magic word" (eg, S.H.A.R.P.).

   ☞ *Some adjustment may be necessary to come up with an intelligible word. Encourage people to change their labels slightly to obtain a more fitting initial letter. Or they could add an extra vowel or consonant to create a memorable magic word.*

2) At the direction of the trainer, participants loudly speak their magic word three times in unison.

3) The trainer asks participants to post this word on themselves and wear it for the remainder of the session.

☞ *They may write it on their name tag, or make a "paper button" to tape or pin on themselves to wear "on their sleeve," etc.*

4) The trainer points out that the magic words have the power of a wizard, to brighten the day. Several times throughout the remainder of the session/workshop, the trainer asks participants to reflect on their "magic word," and by recalling the personal energizers it stands for, to let it rekindle their vitality.

The trainer suggests to participants that they post their magic word conspicuously both at home and at work as a reminder of the vitality that is always readily available to them.

VARIATIONS

■ Participants may be asked to mingle and to describe to others the meaning of, and power behind, their magic word.

■ A small group "button pinning ceremony" could be designed as a closing ritual. The "magic words" would be commissioned and celebrated together by the group.

■ This exercise could be combined with, and used as the closing summary for, other positive perception and mental self-care exercises such as *The Power of Positive Thinking* (**Wellness 2**, p 72) or *Drainers and Energizers* (**Stress 3**, p 26).

106 STANDING OVATION

This affirming energizer adds to the positive spirit of a seminar as participants periodically request and receive enthusiastic standing ovations.

GOALS

To help people learn to ask for and receive affirmation.

To promote a high energy level and positive group spirit.

GROUP SIZE

Best with large groups; does not work as well with groups smaller than 25.

TIME FRAME

3 minutes

PROCESS

1) The trainer points out that all too often in life, when we do good things for others, our contributions are not recognized—at least publicly. He tells the group that they are about to remedy this oversight.

2) The trainer asks, "Who in this room would like to be recognized and affirmed publicly?" One participant volunteer is selected to come forward.

   The trainer asks the volunteer to tell the group her name and something positive about herself. When she has finished, the trainer instructs the group to rise and give her a tumultuous standing ovation, with applause, cheers, whistles—the works!

3) The trainer informs the group that anyone who wishes may receive a standing ovation at anytime throughout the day. He goes on to outline the procedure:

   ➤ Simply stand and request a standing ovation for yourself by shouting, "I want a standing ovation!"

   ➤ No matter what else is going on in the room at the time, the entire group will rise to its feet and provide the ovation.

   ➤ You may not request a standing ovation for someone else. To receive a standing ovation, you must ask for it yourself.

☞ *You may want to be sure that while you're giving these guidelines, one or two people request standing ovations. This will prime the pump and encourage people to join in. If no one makes the request encourage them by saying, "Hey, doesn't someone else want an ovation now?" or "Let's do a couple more, now that we're warmed up. Who else wants one?"*

4) Throughout the remainder of the seminar whenever someone asks for an ovation, the leader enthusiastically leads the cheering. If the energy in the room dwindles, the trainer may encourage others to make the request, or may set up a few "plants" during a break.

TRAINER'S NOTES

*We first experienced this process with Matt Weinstein, author of **Playfair**. Since then we've seen it used by many others. We don't know who originally created this exercise. But, whoever you are, wherever you are, rise right now and ask for your ovation. We cheer you!! It's a great idea.*

©1994 Whole Person Press 210 W Michigan Duluth MN 55802   (800) 247-6789

107 WAVES

In this relaxing interlude, participants take turns impersonating the undulating movement of seaweed being washed over by waves.

GOALS

To let go, relax and feel the rhythm and support of other people.

TIME FRAME

5–10 minutes

PROCESS

1) The trainer asks participants to join with two other people to form a trio for this unusual relaxation routine. Trios spread out around the room so that there is plenty of elbow room.

2) Trios decide which person is **Sand, Surf** and **Seaweed.**

   The trainer announces that participants will take turns impersonating stalks of seaweed, anchored to the ocean floor and gently undulating as the waves wash over. She asks a trio to demonstrate as she describes the process.

   ➤ The **Seaweed** person in each group should stand in front of the **Sand** and the **Surf** partners, facing away, with feet about 12" apart. Let your hands rest at your sides and relax as much as possible.

   🖝 *Be sure to point out that the purpose of this exercise is relaxation—so laughter, rough-housing or scare tactics are inappropriate. No "Jaws" allowed—the person in the middle needs to be able to trust the other partners!*

   ➤ The **Sand** and **Surf** partners should take a position behind and on either side of **Seaweed** so that you can support him when he leans back slightly. Put one hand on **Seaweed's** shoulder and the other in the midback area. Be sure your own feet are firmly planted, one in front of the other, to brace yourself for holding his weight.

   ➤ **Seaweeds** should start to rock or sway slowly and gently from side to side against the pressure of the others' hands. Gradually, you should relinquish control and relax as you allow the other two to push you gently back and forth.

☞ *Caution participants not to make any abrupt movements or lean the person too far forward or backward. The motion should be like a gentle swaying or circular movement.*

The person in the middle should keep his legs and torso straight, letting his whole body sway as a unit and rocking from heel to toe as he relaxes into the undulating motion.

3) The trainer clarifies the instructions as needed and invites trios to "make waves" with **Seaweed** in the middle.

☞ *The impact of this experience is enhanced if participants visualize the seaweed and ocean image. Encourage people to use all their senses as aids to the relaxation process.*

4) After about 2 minutes, the trainer interrupts and asks participants to exchange roles—the **Sand** person goes to the middle this time. The instructions from *Step 2* are repeated so that the other partners can assume the correct position for making waves.

☞ *You may want to repeat the cautions—especially if you noticed any problems during the first round.*

5) After about 2 minutes, the trainer again calls time and invites the **Surf** person in each trio to take a turn in the waves.

Submitted by Krysta Eryn Kavenaugh.

108 WEATHER REPORT

In pairs, participants simulate meteorological phenomena as they ex-change back rubs.

GOALS

To release muscular tension in neck, shoulders and back.

To enhance relaxation through imagery.

GROUP SIZE

Unlimited, as long as there is space for dyads to spread out.

TIME FRAME

5–10 minutes for each partner.

PROCESS

1) The trainer invites participants to pair up with a neighbor for a revitalizing meteorological experiment. As soon as everyone has a partner, dyads are instructed to decide who is a **winter** and who is a **summer.**

   ☞ *Be sure everyone has a partner. If there is an uneven number in the group, you get to participate, too!*

2) The trainer instructs the **summer** person in each pair to sit down in a chair. The**winter** person is directed to stand behind and place her hands on *summer's* shoulders.

   As soon as everyone is in position, the trainer guides the **winters** in massaging the head, neck and shoulders of their *summer* partners, using the images and instructions in the **Weather Report** script to describe the process.

   ☞ *Demonstrate the techniques as you describe them. Encourage receiving partners to give feedback with appreciative sighs, groans and exclamations—and to report any discomfort. Givers adjust their technique accordingly.*

3) Partners exchange positions and *Step 2* is repeated, with the trainer guiding **summers** through the massage of their *winter* partners.

©1994 Whole Person Press 210 W Michigan Duluth MN 55802   (800) 247-6789

WEATHER REPORT Script

SNOWFLAKES

> *Begin by tapping your fingers lightly along your partner's shoulders. Gradually extend these gently falling* **snowflakes** *up the back of your partner's neck and then to the top of the head.*

RAINDROPS

> *Now move back to the shoulders and turn those snowflakes into* **raindrops** *tapping a little harder across the shoulders, up the neck and all over the scalp.*

HAILSTONES

> *Return again to the shoulders and pretend your fingers are* **hailstones,** *cascading down out of the sky. Flick your wrists and tap harder all over the shoulder, head and neck area.*

THUNDER

> *Now use the* **thunder** *stroke massaging the same area. Cup your hands and clap them across the shoulders and down along the top of the arms.*

LIGHTNING

> *Next comes the* **lightning.** *Use the sides of your hands and a chopping motion to pound the large muscles of the shoulders and upper back. Try different intensities. Check with your partner to find out what pressure feels good.*

TORNADO

> *Massage the whole neck and shoulder area with thumbs. Press deep into the muscle and rub in circles that resemble the eye of a* **tornado.**

METEOR SHOWER

> *Now make fists and pound down the back on either side of the column. Adjust the intensity of this* **meteor shower** *to your partner's liking.*

TIDAL WAVE

> *Return now to the starting position for the* **tidal wave.** *Place your palms on top of your partner's shoulders and use the heel of your hand to move the muscles of the shoulders back and forth like kneading bread.*

©1994 Whole Person Press 210 W Michigan Duluth MN 55802   (800) 247-6789

CALM

*Again return to the starting position. Place your palms firmly on top of your partner's shoulders and rest quietly as the **calm** after a storm. Send warmth into the muscles as you imagine energy flowing out of your hands and into your partner's shoulders.*

Now lift your hands several inches above your partner's shoulders and wait a few seconds. Then lower your hands to your side and shake them gently.

Submitted by Martha Belknap.

©1994 Whole Person Press 210 W Michigan Duluth MN 55802   (800) 247-6789

Resources

GUIDE TO THE RESOURCES SECTION

This resources section is intended to provide assistance for planning and preparation as you develop and expand your wellness training and health promotion consulting in various settings.

TIPS FOR TRAINERS p. 136

Suggestions for designing a multi-session course or workshop using the exercises in **Structured Exercises in Wellness Promotion Volume 3**.

EDITORS' CHOICE p. 139

Recommendations from the editors on their favorite exercises from **Wellness 3** and hints for on-the-job wellness training.

> Four****Star Exercises: The Best of **Wellness 3** p. 139
> Especially for the Workplace p. 141

WINNING COMBINATIONS p. 143

Outlines for sessions of varying length using exercises from **Wellness 3** in combination. Plus notes on natural companion processes from other **Structured Exercises** volumes.

> Whole Person Wellness Presentation Plus (45–90 minutes)
> Healthy Eating Habits Mini-Workshop ($1^1/_4$–$2^1/_2$ hours)

ANNOTATED INDEXES to Wellness 3 p. 145

Guides to specific content segments and group activities incorporated in exercises from **Wellness 3**, identified by page reference, time frame, brief description, and comments on use.

> Index to CHALKTALKS p. 145
> Index to DEMONSTRATIONS p. 147
> Index to PHYSICAL ENERGIZERS p. 148
> Index to MENTAL ENERGIZERS p. 149
> Index to RELAXATION ROUTINES p. 149

CONTRIBUTORS/EDITORS p. 150

Data on trainers who have shared their best process ideas in this volume. All are highly skilled educators and most provide in-house training, consultation, or workshops that may be valuable to you in planning comprehensive wellness programs. Many contributors are also established authors of well-respected materials on stress, wellness, and training issues.

WHOLE PERSON PUBLICATIONS p. 155

Descriptions of trainer-tested audio, video, and print resources available from the stress and wellness specialists.

TIPS FOR TRAINERS

Designing a Multi-Session Course or Workshop Using Structured Exercises in Wellness Promotion Volume 3

One-shot wellness presentations can be fun and motivating, but if you are interested in helping people make significant behavior change, you will need to plan an extended learning experience with skill practice during and between sessions, opportunities for mid-course evaluation and corrections, and lots of personal and interpersonal support. There are several effective models for longer learning experiences.

- **Course with 4–8 Sessions**. (6–16 hours)
  This typical adult education model often features weekly meetings of 90 minutes to 2 hours and offers maximum responsiveness to participant needs as the trainer adjusts the course content and process from week to week to meet the expressed concerns of the group. Participants have an opportunity to implement and practice new behaviors between sessions and report back regularly on progress.

- **One- or Two-Day Workshop**. (8–16 hours)
  The workshop setting allows larger blocks of time to develop key concepts, explore options, and make connections. This model tends to build group camaraderie quickly, without wasting time getting reacquainted and warmed up before each session. Unfortunately, there is no between-session opportunity for reflection and experimentation.

- **Combination Workshop/Course**. (9–20 hours)
  Start with a half-day or full-day exploratory and goal-setting workshop (4–8 hours) with a 3–6 session follow-up. This model creates enough shared experience initially to solidify the group, yet still allows you to incorporate participant's individual goals in planning the remaining sessions.

Any of these models can work well. Choose the one that fits your setting, audience and personal style. We have designed the **Structured Exercises** volumes to give you the resources you need, no matter what model you choose. The **Whole Person Wellness Presentation Plus** outline on page 142 makes a good starting point for designing a multi-session course. Use the **Personal Wellness Wheel** (p. 17) or **Health Lifelines** (p. 37) for the first session. Compile suggestions from participants on their personal goals, then choose themes for the remaining sessions that address these issues. You may want to supplement the exercises in this volume with thematic processes from other **Structured Exercises** volumes.

No matter what the model, in designing a wellness course or longer workshop, you need to incorporate all the content objectives in a sequence that takes advantage of the extended time period and flows naturally over the sessions,

©1994 Whole Person Press 210 W Michigan Duluth MN 55802   (800) 247-6789

using processes that activate and reinforce healthy group dynamics. At the same time, you need to create each individual session with its own objectives and rhythm that maximizes participant involvement.

● Begin with a welcoming icebreaker that helps people get acquainted and introduces some aspect of the course content. The **Icebreakers** section of every **Structured Exercises** volume has several topical warm-ups.

● Present the major content segment of the session. In the early part of the course, this may come from the **Wellness Exploration** section of **Structured Exercises**.

As the course progresses, you will want to focus on practical applications like those presented in the **Self-Care Strategies** section. Every volume of **Structured Exercises** includes in this section processes addressing physical (fitness, nutrition, relaxation), mental, emotional, spiritual, lifestyle, and self-care issues. Choose several that fit the goals of your group, and plan sessions around them, using related icebreakers, planning processes, and group energizers.

● Schedule in time for personal reflection and application of the concepts you've presented. Nearly every **Structured Exercise** gives you a worksheet or handout to help people focus. Then be sure to allow time for sharing in small groups. This is really the heart of the learning process, the place where people test out their insights, clarify their goals, and learn from others.

● Every session should end with a concrete planning or application process where participants identify goals and next steps. Many of the designs in **Structured Exercises** have built-in closure processes, but you might want to check out the variety of options in the **Planning/Closure** sections.

● In a multi-session course, or between workshop days, be sure to assign some homework. This could take the form of skill practice, journaling, or tracking behaviors as outlined in **Daily Wellness Graph** (p. 100). Remember that it's what happens at home that will be the real measure of your success.

● Do take time at the end of every segment to summarize and provide transition. Polling the group for insights is a great way to do this. It gives people a chance to reinforce their learning, adds to the corporate wisdom, and gives you a final opportunity to fill in the gaps.

● Don't forget to check out the **Group Energizers** section for demonstrations and activities that can vividly illustrate key concepts and provide a change of pace.

● If relaxation/meditation skills are important to your agenda, teach a different type at every session and encourage participants to practice in between.

Or teach one key technique and practice it at every session.

At the final session of your course/workshop, take time to celebrate what you have shared together. **Health Report Cards** (p. 109) allows participants an opportunity to give positive feedback on progress. **Fortune Cookies** (p. 106) is a more whimsical affirmation of best wishes for wellness.

As you plan, it's helpful to think in time modules, and then use these modules as mix and match building blocks. We tend to conceptualize in 45 minute blocks and many of the processes in the **Structured Exercises** volumes use this time frame. It's just about the time you'll need to introduce a concept, ask participants to reflect and apply it to their own life, and facilitate small group sharing to compare notes and receive support—with a few moments to elicit summary comments and insights. Toss in a group energizer or two, and you have an hour block. Icebreakers and planning processes usually take about 20 minutes, or half a module. Some of the extended reflection exercises and creative explorations take up to 90 minutes, or two modules. Start with a key exercise or two for each session, then supplement with other processes until you fill time blocks.

A Note on Group Dynamics

At the beginning of each session, participants will need time to regroup, touch base, focus. During the first few sessions, use a structured approach to this warm-up time with a thematic icebreaker such as **My Mother Says** (p. 1), **Part of Me** (p. 10), **Getting to Know You** (p. 12), **Galloping Gourmet** (p. 14), **Well Cards** (p. 32), or **Sabotage and Self-Care** (p. 2).

In later sessions simple check-in "rounds" (eg, homework report, progress on goals) will work well. For efficiency and bonding you may want to use a buddy system where participants pair and share at the beginning of each meeting. Switch the pairings a couple of times during the course.

As people get to know each other better, you will need to allocate more time during the sessions for interaction. People will be eager to tell their success stories and to hear how others are doing. As respect for each other grows, participants will also ask for advice or encouragement.

©1994 Whole Person Press 210 W Michigan Duluth MN 55802   (800) 247-6789

EDITORS' CHOICE

Although all 36 exercises in this volume are practical, creative, and time- tested, we must admit that we use some more often than others. When people call us and ask for suggestions about which exercises to incorporate into their workshop designs, we typically recommend some of our favorites—processes that have worked over and over again with many audiences, readings and activities that are guaranteed to charm a group. We call these our FOUR****STAR choices.

Four**Star Exercise**   **Page**   **Comments (Timing)**

75 Health Oriented People Hunt   Health conscious variation of a classic
                    p. 6   icebreaker gets people mixed up and
                           tuned in. Be sure to regulate the pace so
                           people can discuss the bonus questions.
                           (15–20 min)

79 Personal Wellness Wheel   A memorable model for whole person
                 p. 17   well-being that includes life areas such
                           as vocational and environmental. Solid
                           centerpiece exercise for a 90-minute
                           presentation or longer workshop.
                           (15–20 min)

83 Health Lifelines   p. 37   This revealing projective exercise allows
                           lots of latitude for people to uncover and
                           tackle issues of concern to them.
                           (75–90 min)

84 Stand Up and Be Counted   Bill Hettler's action-packed quiz is terrific
                 p. 44   for a large group that doesn't know each
                           other. The process also helps you get a
                           sense of your audience and their issues.
                           (15–20 min)

87 Consciousness-Raising Diet   Family physician Grant Christopher's
                 p. 60   memorable questions heighten aware-
                           ness of eating attitudes—the first step
                           towards healthy change in behaviors.
                           (10–15 min)

88 Countdown to Relaxation   Nancy's favorite mental break and
                 p. 62   insomnia prescription. (5–10 min)

90 Journal to Music   p. 70   Powerful tool for well-being. Use it in a
                           session or for homework. The results can
                           be private or public, often profound. Music
                           truly enhances the experience. See
                           variations for suggestions on adapting the

process to fit your group and content areas. (60–90)

91 Openness and Intimacy
p. 76

Sharing thoughts and feelings is an essential skill for nurturing mental and interpersonal well-being. This classic process uses the fishbowl technique for observing and giving feedback on communication styles. (50–60 min)

93 Footloose and Fancy Free
p. 86

Don's favorite fantasy technique for uncovering hidden values and motivations. Or maybe it's just his favorite fantasy of freedom! This self-care consciousness-raiser can be used alone or in combination with a specific goal-setting process. (10–20 min)

94 Polaroid Perspectives
p. 90

An unusual metaphor prompts reflection on progress to date and stimulates an attitude of self-responsibility for future development. Use for progress reports in a multi-session course. Requires Polaroid camera. (30–50 min)

102 Limericks
p. 120

Nancy loves this light-hearted counterpoint to the typical heavy-duty themes of wellness courses, but it's not for every group. Save it for folks who appreciate and enjoy the creative process. And don't forget the rhyming dictionary! (15–20 min)

©1994 Whole Person Press 210 W Michigan Duluth MN 55802   (800) 247-6789

ESPECIALLY FOR THE WORKPLACE

Most of the exercises in this volume are "generic" wellness processes that can be easily adapted to a variety of settings. When you are asked to conduct on-site health promotion programs, you may want to select content or processes that are particularly applicable in the workplace. All of the exercises listed below should be appropriate in nearly any job setting.

Workplace Exercise	Page	Comments (Timing)
76 Part of Me	p. 10	Participant use items brought from home to introduce themselves and to reflect on the underlying values that influence their self-care choices. Works well with an intact staff who always learns more about each other in this process. Also effective in team-building experiences. (2–3 min per person)
80 Wellness Culture Test	p. 22	Participants analyze the "corporate culture" using Don Ardell's clever quiz, then take steps to reshape group norms in a health-enhancing direction. An opportunity to gripe and to take action. (60–90 min)
81 Pathology of Normalcy	p. 29	A perfect companion to the Wellness Culture Test, this satirical reading from Earl Hipp highlights the absurdity of what's "normal." Really hits home. (5 min)
92 That's the Spirit	p. 82	Keith Sehnert's spiritual checkup goes beyond religion to highlight values-based actions that can enrich well-being. An inoffensive, effective tool for raising these important issues in the workplace. (10–15 min)
95 Closing Statements	p. 97	Simple process that prompts people to focus on what they have gained from the experience. Don't miss the pairing and sharing techniques in the Variations. (10–30 min)
96 Daily Wellness Graph	p. 100	Systematic tool for setting whole person wellness goals and charting progress. Especially useful as part of a several-week course. (20–30 min, then 5 min daily)

©1994 Whole Person Press 210 W Michigan Duluth MN 55802   (800) 247-6789

WINNING COMBINATIONS

Whole Person Wellness Presentation Plus (45–90 minutes)

Exercise 79, **Personal Wellness Wheel** (p. 17, 15–20 min) is an excellent centerpiece for any wellness presentation. The eight dimensions of well-being allow for affirmation as well as confrontation about wellness patterns and areas of concern.

Follow up this general assessment with one or more thematic self-care processes that you anticipate will be important to your audience.

- **Physical**: Exercise 85, **Auto/Body Checkup** (p. 49, 15–20 min); **Fit To Be Interviewed**, Exercise 89 (p. 65, 45 min); **Consciousness-Raising Diet** (p. 60, 10–15 min).

- **Social**: Exercise 75, **Health Oriented People Hunt** (p. 6, 15—20 min), substituting attributes and questions that highlight interpersonal well-being issues; Exercise 91, **Openness and Intimacy** (p. 76, 50–60 min).

- **Vocational**: Exercise 56, **Compass** (Wellness 3, 30–60 min), helps put work into context; **Job Motivators**, Exercise 128 (Wellness 4, 40–45 min), explores the meaning of work.

- **Environmental**: Ardell's **Wellness Culture Test**, Exercise 80 (p. 22, 60–90 min) looks at the immediate environment and could be extended to a more global perspective.

- **Psychological**: Exercise 94, **Polaroid Perspectives** (p. 90, 30–50 min), provides a developmental perspective; Exercise 86, **Chemical Independence** (p. 55, 25–35 min), explores addictive patterns.

- **Spiritual**: Exercise 92, **That's the Spirit** (p. 82, 10–15 min).

- **Intellectual**: Exercise 99, **50 Excuses for a Closed Mind** (p. 113, 5–15 min), could be expanded to include a presentation/discussion on nurturing a lively mind.

- **Emotional**: Exercise 90, **Journal to Music** (p. 70, 60–90 min), could be used for exploring emotional well-being; Exercise 101, **Feelings Factory** (p. 118, 2–3 min), is a related group energizer; **Self-Esteem Grid**, Exercise 123 (Wellness 4, 45–50 min), looks at another component of mental health.

Add appropriate group energizers as desired, and finish with Exercise 95, **Closing Statements** (p. 97, 10–30 min) or for a multi-session course, **Health Report Cards**, Exercise 98 (p. 109, 25–30 min).

Healthy Eating Habits Mini-Workshop ($1^1/_4 - 2^1/_2$ hours)

You will no doubt be asked at some point, and perhaps often, to provide a session or workshop targeting the "shame and blame" issues of wellness: physical fitness, chemical use (alcohol/tobacco/drugs), nutrition/eating habits/weight control. Since our general bias is to always present wellness in the whole person context, we would encourage you to start with a general wellness assessment like **Health Lifelines**, Exercise 83 (p. 37, 75–90 minutes) or the **Personal Wellness Wheel**, Exercise 79 (p. 17, 15–20 minutes) that allows participants to consider these problematic areas in relationship to wider health and wholeness concerns, balanced with their self-care strengths and positive behaviors.

This volume includes several non-judgmental exercises that can be grouped together as a mini-workshop on eating patterns that applies not only to the overweight. Start with **My Mother Says,** Exercise 73A (p. 1, 10–15 min), inviting participants to focus on food and eating-related messages they heard in their childhood and adolescence. This personal exploration and sharing should level the playing field. Then break up into small groups and analyze the nutritional value and calorie count of a favorite meal using **Galloping Gourmet**, Exercise 78 (p. 14, 20–30 min). Follow this eye-opening experience with Dr Christopher's **Consciousness-Raising Diet**, Exercise 87 (p. 60, 10–15 minutes), with it's five memorable questions.

Include some energy breaks like the empowering **Breathing Elements**, Exercise 100 (p. 116, 5 min), or the supportive **Waves**, Exercise 107 (p. 130, 5–10 min). Exercise 33, **Noontime Energizers** (Wellness 1, 5–10 min), with its emphasis on identifying and satisfying all types of hungers might be an enlightening addition if you have time.

The icebreaker **Sabotage and Self-Care**, Exercise 73B (p. 2, 10–15 min), can be easily transformed into a thoughtful closing exercise that allows folks to acknowledge the difficulty of sustaining new patterns. Or use Exercise 95, **Closing Statements** (p. 97, 10–30 min), which is generic enough to stimulate sharing of positive insights as well as planning for problem-oriented behavior change. If you'd rather end on a less serious note, try **Fortune Cookies**, Exercise 97 (p. 106, 15–20 min).

©1994 Whole Person Press 210 W Michigan Duluth MN 55802   (800) 247-6789

ANNOTATED INDEXES

Index to CHALKTALKS

©1994 Whole Person Press 210 W Michigan Duluth MN 55802   (800) 247-6789

Index to DEMONSTRATIONS

Index to PHYSICAL ENERGIZERS

©1994 Whole Person Press 210 W Michigan Duluth MN 55802   (800) 247-6789

Index to MENTAL ENERGIZERS

Index to RELAXATION ROUTINES

©1994 Whole Person Press 210 W Michigan Duluth MN 55802   (800) 247-6789

CONTRIBUTORS

Donald B Ardell, Director, Wellness Institute, University of Central Florida, Orlando FL 32816. 407/823-2453. Don is the author of the landmark book **High Level Wellness: An Alternative To Doctors, Drugs, and Disease** and ten other books, including **Die Healthy** and **Freedom, Self-Management, and the Wellness Orgasm** (with Grant Donovan). He also publishes the quarterly **Ardell Wellness Report**, of which there are now 33 editions in print. (for a sample copy send a SASE to Dr Ardell).

Kent D Beeler, EdD. 6025 Compton Street, Indianapolis IN 46220-2003. 317/259-8064. Kent is an active advocate of wellness at the college and university level. His experiential workshops have been popular with campus and professional groups interested in personal lifestyle promotion. Kent is a year-round, recreational runner, and has served on the Directorate Body, American College Personnel Assoc Comm VIII: Wellness.

Martha Belknap, MA. 1170 Dixon Road, Gold Hill, Boulder CO 80302. 303/447-9642. Marti is an educational consultant with a specialty in creative relaxation and stress management skills. She has 30 years of teaching experience at all levels. Marti offers relaxation workshops and creativity courses through schools, universities, hospitals and businesses. She is the author of **Taming Your Dragons**, a book and cassette tape of creative relaxation activities for home and school.

Grant Christopher, MD. Bemidji Clinic, 12333 4th St NW, Bemidji MN 56601. 218/751-1280 (w). Grant is a board certified family physician who practices and promotes the philosophy of wellness personally and professionally in his medical practice and through the teaching of seminars on wellness.

Lyman Coleman, MDiv, PhD. Serendipity House, Box 1012, Littleton CO 80160. 303/798-1313. Founder and director of Serendipity Workshops, Lyman has spent the past 30 years training over 150,000 church leaders of all denominations in small group processes. Author of scores of books, including a small group discussion version of the Bible, Lyman's innovative approach combines Bible study, group building and values orientation with personal story telling.

Joel Goodman, EdD. Director, The HUMOR Project, 110 Spring Street, Saratoga Springs NY 12866. 518/587-8770. Joel is a popular speaker, consultant and seminar leader who has presented to over 500,000 corporate managers, health care leaders, educators, and other helping professionals throughout the U.S. and abroad. Author of 8 books, Joel publishes **Laughing Matters** magazine and HUMOResources mail order bookstore catalog, and sponsors the annual international conference on "The Positive Power of Humor and Creativity."

©1994 Whole Person Press 210 W Michigan Duluth MN 55802   (800) 247-6789

Bill Hettler, MD. President of Lifestyle Improvement Programs and Systems, 718 Linwood Avenue, Stevens Point WI 54481. 715/345-1735. Bill is a phy-sician educator who has spent his professional life developing health promotion systems and materials. He is a co-founder of the National Wellness Institute. Bill was also the originator of the **National Wellness Conference** and has been an active contributor to both professional and popular publications. For the past ten years, he has been active in developing computer software to assist people in making positive health changes.

Earl Hipp, Human Resource Development Inc, 333 Washington Ave North, Suite 300, Minneapolis MN 55401. 612/349-2717. Earl is the president of Human Resource Development Inc, a management consulting and training firm special-izing in individual and organizational change resilience.

David R Johnson, MN, RN. St Francis College, 2701 Spring Street, Fort Wayne IN 46808. 219/434-3234 (w). David is an assistant professor of Nursing at St Francis College as well as an employee assistance specialist and certified marriage and family therapist with the Lindenview Counseling Center in Ft Wayne IN. He presents various community and corporate workshops whose topics include stress management, leadership, chemical dependency, self-esteem, grief, team building, and motivation.

Krysta Eryn Kavenaugh, MA, CSP. 955 Lake Drive, St Paul MN 55120. 800/829-8437 (w) 612/725-6763 (h). Krysta is a speaker, trainer, and consultant. Her mission is to take people "into the heart of wisdom." She speaks with style, substance, and spirit. She is also the managing editor of **Marriage** magazine. Her favorite keynote topic is "Romancing Yourself: Taking Care of You is Taking Care of Business." She also speaks on proactive support teams, turning adversity to our advantage, ecology, and customized business topics.

Merrill Kempfert, MDiv. Community Relations Representative, Heights Psychi-atric Hospital, 103 Hospital Loop NE, Albuquerque NM 87109, 505/883-3589 (w) 505/897-6325 (h). As a Lutheran pastor and one who works in the addiction field, Merrill struggles with leading a balanced life, juggling work, family and outdoor interests.

Jean Mershon, Employee Development Specialist and Wellness Coordinator, St Louis County. Room 202, 100 N 5th Ave W, Duluth MN 55802. 218/726-2446. Jean coordinates employee development and training for 2400 county employ-ees. The wellness program offers a wide variety of health promotion programs and activities for county employees.

Sandy Queen, Director, LIFEWORKS, PO Box 2668, Columbia MD 21045. 401/796-5310. Sandy is the founder and director of Lifeworks Inc, a training/counseling firm that specializes in helping people take a better look at their lives through humor, laughter, and play. Author of **Wellness Activities for Youth**, she has developed many innovative programs in the areas of stress-reduction, humor, children's wellness, and self-esteem.

©1994 Whole Person Press 210 W Michigan Duluth MN 55802   (800) 247-6789

Ann Raber, Director, Mennonite Mutual Aid Wellness Program, 1110 N Main Box 483, Goshen IN 46526. 219/533-9511. Mennonite Mutual Aid offers wellness programs for both adults and children. The sessions incorporate a Christian perspective, emphasizing the wholeness of the individual. The programs utilize active participation, small support groups, and local leadership. MMA also provides discussion guides for groups to study advanced directives, AIDS, Health Care Reform, and Medical Ethics.

Ronda J Salge, MA, RMT-BC. 5465 N 650 E Churubus IN 46723. 219/693-9722 (h). As a music therapist, Ronda runs a private practice working with children. She has worked in acute adult psychiatric rehabilitation services, supervision of music therapy practicum experiences and providing adult mentally retarded/developmentally disabled habilitation services. Ronda conducts workshops for community and professional groups on "Journaling with Music" and "Relaxation Techniques with Music."

Marcia A Schnorr, RN EdD. Nursing Instructor, Kishwaukee College, Rt 38 & Malta Rd, Malta IL 60150. 815/825-2086 (w) 815/562-6823 (h). Marcia is the parish nurse of St Paul Lutheran Church, Rochelle IL, 815/562-2744, coordinator of the Lutheran Church-Missouri Synod Parish Nurse Ministry, and an adjunct professor in parish nursing for Concordia University in Wisconsin.

Keith W Sehnert, MD. 4210 Fremont Avenue South, Minneapolis MN 55409. 612/920-0102 (w), 612/824-5134 (h). Keith is a family doctor who has become a leader in the medical self-care movement. He spends much energy in print (**How To Be Your Own Doctor—Sometimes**, **Stress/Unstress** and **Self-care/ Wellcare**), and in person, urging people to improve their physical, mental and spiritual well-being. He has an independent practice in St Louis Park MN.

David X Swenson, PhD. Assoc Professor of Management, College of St Scholastica, 1200 Kenwood Ave, Duluth MN 55811. 218/723-6476 (w) 218/ 724-6903 (h). A licensed consulting psychologist, Dave maintains a private practice in addition to his educational and therapeutic roles at the college. He provides consultation and training to human services, health and law enforcement agencies and is the author of **Stress Management in the Criminal Justice System.** Dave also develops stress management software.

Mark Warner, EdD. Assistant Vice president for Human Resources and Facility Management, James Madison University, Harrisonburg VA 22807. 703/568-3685. In addition to his administrative duties, Mark teaches, consults, writes, and presents on the topics of wellness promotion, leadership development, and organizational development.

FUTURE CONTRIBUTORS

If you have developed an exciting, effective structured exercise you'd like to share with other trainers in the field of stress or wellness, please send it to us for consideration, using the following guidelines:

- Your entry should be written in a format similar to those in this volume.

- Contributors must either guarantee that the materials they submit are not previously copyrighted or provide a copyright release for inclusion in the Whole Person **Structured Exercises** series.

- When you have adapted the work of others, please acknowledge the original source of ideas or activities.

©1994 Whole Person Press 210 W Michigan Duluth MN 55802   (800) 247-6789

EDITORS

All exercises in this volume not specifically attributed to other contributors are the creative efforts of the editors, who have been designing, collecting, and experimenting with structured processes in their teaching, training and consultation work since the late 1960s.

Nancy Loving Tubesing, EdD, holds a masters degree in group counseling and a doctorate in counselor education. She served as editor of the *Society for Wholistic Medicine's* monograph series and articulated the principles of whole person health care in the monograph, **Philosophical Assumptions**. Faculty Associate and Product Development Coordinator at Whole Person Associates, Nancy is always busy compiling and testing teaching designs for future **Structured Exercises** volumes.

Donald A Tubesing, MDiv, PhD, designer of the classic **Stress Skills** seminar and author of the best-selling **Kicking Your Stress Habits**, has been a pioneer in the movement to reintegrate body, mind, and spirit in health care delivery. With his entrepreneurial spirit and background in theology, psychology, and education, Don brings the whole person perspective to his writing, speaking, and consultation in business and industry, government agencies, health care, and human service systems.

Nancy and Don have collaborated on many writing projects over the years, beginning with a small-group college orientation project in 1970 and including two self-help books on whole person wellness, **The Caring Question** (Minneapolis: Augsburg, 1983) and **Seeking Your Healthy Balance** (Duluth: Whole Person Press, 1991), and a score of unusual relaxation audiotapes.

The Tubesings have specialized in developing creative stress management programs and packages for client groups such as the national YMCA (8-session course, **The Y's Way to Stress Management**) and Aid Association for Lutherans (**The Stress Kit** multimedia resource for families).

Their most recent efforts have been directed toward combining the process-oriented approach of the **Structured Exercises** series with the power of video. The resulting three six-session interactive video courses, **WellAware**, **Manage It!**, and **Managing Job Stress**, include participant booklets with worksheets that stimulate personal reflection and application of principles to specific situations, as well as a step-by-step leader manual for guiding group interaction.

©1994 Whole Person Press 210 W Michigan Duluth MN 55802   (800) 247-6789

WORKSHOPS-IN-A-BOOK

KICKING YOUR STRESS HABITS:
A Do-it-yourself Guide to Coping with Stress
Donald A. Tubesing, PhD

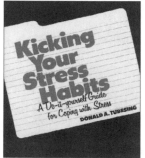

Over a quarter of a million people have found ways to deal with their everyday stress by using **Kicking Your Stress Habits**. This workshop-in-a-book actively involves the reader in assessing stressful patterns and developing more effective coping strategies with helpful "Stop and Reflect" sections in each chapter.

The 10-step planning process and 20 skills for managing stress make **Kicking Your Stress Habits** an ideal text for stress management classes in many different settings, from hospitals to universities and for a wide variety of groups.

❑ **K / Kicking Your Stress Habits / 14.95**

SEEKING YOUR HEALTHY BALANCE:
A Do-it-yourself Guide to Whole Person Well-being
Donald A. Tubesing, PhD and Nancy Loving Tubesing, EdD

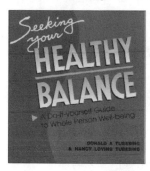

Where can you find the time and energy to "do it all" without sacrificing your health and well-being? **Seeking Your Healthy Balance** helps the reader discover how to make changes toward a more balanced lifestyle by learning effective ways to juggle work, self, and others; clarifying self-care options; and discovering and setting their own personal priorities.

Seeking Your Healthy Balance asks the questions and helps readers find their own answers.

❑ **HB / Seeking Your Healthy Balance / 14.95**

©1994 Whole Person Press 210 W Michigan Duluth MN 55802   (800) 247-6789

STRUCTURED EXERCISES
IN STRESS MANAGEMENT—VOLUMES 1-4
Nancy Loving Tubesing, EdD and Donald A. Tubesing, PhD, Editors

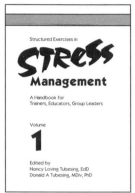

Each book in this four-volume series contains 36 ready-to-use teaching modules that involve the participant—as a whole person—in learning how to manage stress more effectively.

Each exercise is carefully designed by top stress-management professionals. Instructions are clearly written and field-tested so that even beginning trainers can smoothly lead a group through warm-up and closure, reflection and planning, and action and interaction—all with minimum preparation time.

Each Stress Handbook is brimming with practical ideas that you can weave into your own teaching designs or mix and match to develop new programs for varied settings, audiences, and time frames. In each volume you'll find **Icebreakers, Stress Assessments, Management Strategies, Skill Builders, Action Planners, Closing Processes** and **Group Energizers**—all with a special focus on stress management.

STRUCTURED EXERCISES
IN WELLNESS PROMOTION—VOLUMES 1-4
Nancy Loving Tubesing, EdD and Donald A. Tubesing, PhD, Editors

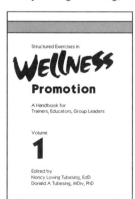

Discover the Wellness Handbooks—from the wellness pioneers at Whole Person Associates. Each volume in this innovative series includes 36 experiential learning activities that focus on whole person health—body, mind, spirit, emotions, relationships, and lifestyle.

The exercises, developed by an interdisciplinary pool of leaders in the wellness movement nationwide, actively encourage people to adopt wellness-oriented attitudes and to develop more responsible self-care patterns.

All process designs in the Wellness Handbooks are clearly explained and have been thoroughly field-tested with diverse audiences so that trainers can use them with confidence. **Icebreakers, Wellness Explorations, Self-Care Strategies, Action Planners, Closings** and **Group Energizers** are all ready-to-go—including reproducible worksheets, scripts, and chalktalk outlines—for the busy professional who wants to develop unique wellness programs without spending oodles of time in preparation.

©1994 Whole Person Press 210 W Michigan Duluth MN 55802   (800) 247-6789

STRUCTURED EXERCISES IN STRESS AND WELLNESS ARE AVAILABLE IN TWO FORMATS

LOOSE-LEAF FORMAT (8 1/2" x 11")

The loose-leaf, 3-ring binder format provides you with maximum flexiblity. The binder gives you plenty of room to add your own adaptations, workshop outlines, or notes right where you need them. The index tabs offer quick and easy access to each section of exercises, and the generous margins allow plenty of room for notes. In addition an extra set of the full-size worksheets and handouts are packaged separately for convenient duplication.

SOFTCOVER FORMAT (6" x 9")

The softcover format is a perfect companion to the loose-leaf version. This smaller book fits easily into your briefcase or bag, and the binding has been designed to remain open on your desk or lecturn. Worksheets and handouts can be enlarged and photocopied for distribution to your participants, or you can purchase sets of worksheet masters.

WORKSHEET MASTERS

The Worksheet Masters for the two Structured Exercise series offer full-size (8 1/2" x 11") photocopy masters. All of the worksheets and handouts for each volume are reproduced in easy-to-read print with professional graphics. All you need to do to complete your workshop preparation is run them through a copier.

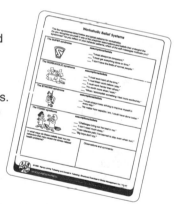

Structured Exercises in Stress Management

- ❑ **Loose-Leaf Edition—Volume 1-4 / $54.95 each**
- ❑ **Softcover Edition—Volume 1-4 / $29.95 each**
- ❑ **Worksheet Masters—Volume 1-4 / $9.95 each**

Structured Exercises in Wellness Promotion

- ❑ **Loose-Leaf Edition—Volume 1-4 / $54.95 each**
- ❑ **Softcover Edition—Volume 1-4 / $29.95 each**
- ❑ **Worksheet Masters—Volume 1-4 / $9.95 each**

©1994 Whole Person Press 210 W Michigan Duluth MN 55802   (800) 247-6789

ADDITIONAL GROUP PROCESS RESOURCES

Our group process exercises are designed to address the whole person—
physical, emotional, mental, spiritual, and social. Developed for trainers by
trainers, all of these group process resources are ready-to-use. The novice
trainer will find everything they need to get started, and the expert trainer will
discover new ideas and concepts to add to their existing programs.

All of the exercises encourage interaction between the leader and the
participants, as well as among the participants. Each exercise includes
everything you need to present a meaningful program: goals, optimal group
size, time frame, materials list, and the complete process instructions.

PLAYFUL ACTIVITIES FOR POWERFUL PRESENTATIONS
Bruce Williamson

This book contains 40 fun exercises designed to fit any group or topic. These
exercises will help you:

- build teamwork
- encourage laughter and playfulness
- relieve stress and tension
- free up the imaginations of participants

> ❏ **PAP / Playful Activities for Powerful Presentations / $19.95**

WORKING WITH GROUPS FROM DYSFUNCTIONAL FAMILIES
Cheryl Hetherington

This collection of 29 proven group activities is designed to heal the pain that
results from growing up in or living in a dysfunctional family. With these
exercises you can:

- promote healing
- build self-esteem
- encourage sharing
- help participants acknowledge their feelings

WORKING WITH GROUPS FROM DYSFUNCTIONAL FAMILIES
REPRODUCIBLE WORKSHEET MASTERS

A complete package of full-size (8 1/2" x 11") photocopy masters that include
all the worksheets and handouts from **Working with Groups from Dysfunctional Families** is available to you. Use the masters for easy duplication of
the handouts for each participant.

> ❏ **DFH / Working with Groups from Dysfunctional Families / $19.95**
> ❏ **DFW / Dysfunctional Families Worksheet Masters / $9.95**

©1994 Whole Person Press 210 W Michigan Duluth MN 55802   (800) 247-6789

WORKING WITH WOMEN'S GROUPS Volumes 1 & 2
Louise Yolton Eberhardt

The two volumes of **Working with Women's Groups** have been completely revised and updated. These exercises will help women explore issues that are of perennial concern as well as today's hot topics.

- consciousness-raising (volume 1)
- self-discovery (volume 1)
- assertiveness training (volume 1)
- sexuality issues (volume 2)
- women of color (volume 2)
- leadership skills training (volume 2)

> ❏ **WG1 / Working with Women's Groups—Volume 1 / $19.95**
> ❏ **WG2 / Working with Women's Groups—Volume 2 / $19.95**

WORKING WITH MEN'S GROUPS
Roger Karsk and Bill Thomas

Also revised and updated, this volume is a valuable resource for anyone working with men's groups. The exercises cover a variety of topics, including:

- self discovery
- parenting
- conflict
- intimacy

> ❏ **MG / Working with Men's Groups / $19.95**

WELLNESS ACTIVITIES FOR YOUTH Volumes 1 & 2
Sandy Queen

Each volume of **Wellness Activities for Youth** helps leaders teach children and teenagers about wellness with an emphasis on FUN. The concepts include:

- values
- stress and coping
- self-esteem
- personal well-being

WELLNESS ACTIVITIES FOR YOUTH WORKSHEET MASTERS
Complete packages of full-size (8 1/2" x 11") photocopy masters that include all the worksheets and handouts from **Wellness Activities for Youth Volumes 1 and 2** are available to you. Use the masters for easy duplication of the handouts for each participant.

> ❏ **WY1 / Wellness Activities for Youth Volume 1 / $19.95**
> ❏ **WY2 / Wellness Activities for Youth Volume 2 / $19.95**
> ❏ **WY1W / Wellness Activities for Youth V.1 Worksheet Masters / $9.95**
> ❏ **WY2W / Wellness Activities for Youth V. 2 Worksheet Masters / $9.95**

RELAXATION AUDIOTAPES

Perhaps you're an old
hand at relaxation, looking
for new ideas. Or maybe
you're a beginner, just
testing the waters.
Whatever your relaxation
needs, Whole Person
tapes provide a whole
family of techniques for
reducing physical and
mental stress. To assist in
your decision-making, you
may want to know more
about different types of
relaxation.

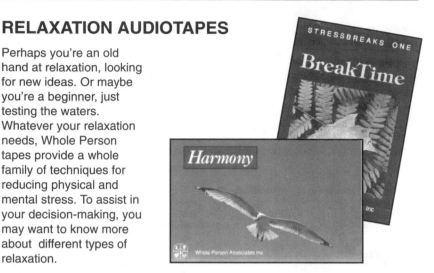

We offer six different types of relaxation techniques in our twenty-one tapes.
The Whole Person series ranges from simple breathing and stretching
exercises, to classic autogenic and progressive relaxation sequences, to
guided meditations and whimsical daydreams. All are carefully crafted to
promote whole person relaxation—body, mind, and spirit. We also provide a
line of music-only tapes, composed specifically for relaxation.

SENSATIONAL RELAXATION

When stress piles up, it becomes a heavy load both physically and emotionally. These full-length relaxation experiences will teach you techniques that
can be used whenever you feel that stress is getting out of control. Choose
one you like and repeat it daily until it becomes second nature then recall that
technique whenever you need it.

> ❏ **CD / Countdown to Relaxation / $9.95**
> ❏ **DS / Daybreak / Sundown / $9.95**
> ❏ **TDB / Take a Deep Breath / $9.95**
> ❏ **RLX / Relax . . . Let Go . . . Relax / $9.95**
> ❏ **SRL / StressRelease / $9.95**
> ❏ **WRM / Warm and Heavy / $9.95**

STRESS BREAKS

Do you need a short energy booster or a quick stress reliever? If you don't
know what type of relaxation you like, or if you are new to guided relaxation
techniques, try one of our Stress Breaks for a quick refocusing or change of
pace any time of the day.

> ❏ **BT / BreakTime / $9.95**
> ❏ **NT / Natural Tranquilizers / $9.95**

©1994 Whole Person Press 210 W Michigan Duluth MN 55802   (800) 247-6789

DAYDREAMS

Escape from the stress around you with guided tours to beautiful places. Picture yourself traveling to the ocean, sitting in a park, luxuriating in the view from the majestic mountains, or enjoying the solitude and serenity of a cozy cabin. The 10-minute escapes included in our Daydream tapes will lead your imagination away from your everyday cares so you can resume your tasks relaxed and comforted.

- ❏ **DD1 / Daydreams 1: Getaways / $9.95**
- ❏ **DD2 / Daydreams 2: Peaceful Places / $9.95**

GUIDED MEDITATION

Take a step beyond relaxation and discover the connection between body and mind with guided meditation. The imagery in our full-length meditations will help you discover your strengths, find healing, make positive life changes, and recognize your inner wisdom.

- ❏ **IH / Inner Healing / $9.95**
- ❏ **PE / Personal Empowering / $9.95**
- ❏ **HBT / Healthy Balancing / $9.95**
- ❏ **SPC / Spiritual Centering / $9.95**

WILDERNESS DAYDREAMS

Discover the healing power of nature with the four tapes in the Wilderness Daydreams series. The eight special journeys will transport you from your harried, stressful surroundings to the peaceful serenity of words and water.

- ❏ **WD1 / Canoe / Rain / $9.95**
- ❏ **WD2 / Island /Spring / $9.95**
- ❏ **WD3 / Campfire / Stream / $9.95**
- ❏ **WD4 / Sailboat / Pond / $9.95**

MUSIC ONLY

No relaxation program would be complete without relaxing melodies that can be played as background to a prepared script or that can be enjoyed as you practice a technique you have already learned. Steven Eckels composed his melodies specifically for relaxation. These "musical prayers for healing" will calm your body, mind, and spirit.

- ❏ **T / Tranquility / $9.95**
- ❏ **H / Harmony / $9.95**
- ❏ **S / Serenity / $9.95**

Titles can be combined for discounts!

QUANTITY DISCOUNT			
1 - 9	10 - 49	50 - 99	100+
$9.95	$8.95	$7.96	CALL

©1994 Whole Person Press 210 W Michigan Duluth MN 55802   (800) 247-6789

RELAXATION RESOURCES

Many trainers and workshop leaders have discovered the benefits of relaxation and visualization in healing the body, mind, and spirit.

30 SCRIPTS FOR RELAXATION, IMAGERY, AND INNER HEALING
Julie Lusk

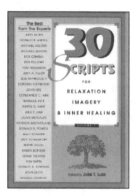

These two volumes are collections of relaxation scripts created by trainers for trainers. The 30 scripts in each of the two volumes have been professionally-tested and fine-tuned so they are ready to use for both novice and expert trainers.

Help your participants change their behavior, enhance their self-esteem, discover inner, private places, and heal themselves through simple trainer-led guided imagery scripts. Both volumes include information on how to use the scripts, suggestions for tailoring them to your specific needs and audience, and information on how to successfully incorporate guided imagery into your existing programs.

❑ **30S / 30 Scripts for Relaxation, Imagery, and Inner Healing—Volume 1 / $19.95**
❑ **30S2 / 30 Scripts for Relaxation, Imagery, and Inner Healing—Volume 2 / $19.95**

INQUIRE WITHIN
Andrew Schwartz

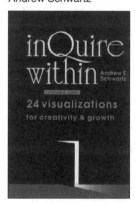

Use visualization to make positive changes in your life. The 24 visualization experiences in **Inquire Within** will help participants enhance their creativity, heal inner pain, learn to relax, and deal with conflict. Each visualization includes questions at the end of the process that encourage deeper reflection and a better understanding of the exercise and the response it invokes.

❑ **IW / Inquire Within / $19.95**

ORDER FORM

Name_____

Address_____

City_____

State/Zip_____

Area Code/Telephone_____

Please make checks payable to:
Whole Person Associates Inc
210 West Michigan
Duluth MN 55802-1908
FAX: 1-218-727-0505
TOLL FREE: 1-800-247-6789

Books / Workshops-In-A-Book

___ Kicking Your Stress Habits .... $14.95 _____

___ Seeking Your Healthy Balance .... $14.95 _____

Structured Exercises in Stress Management Series—Volumes 1-4

___ Stress Softcover Edition .... Vol 1 ___ Vol 2 ___ Vol 3 ___ Vol 4 ___ $29.95 _____

___ Stress Loose-Leaf Edition .... Vol 1 ___ Vol 2 ___ Vol 3 ___ Vol 4 ___ $54.95 _____

___ Stress Worksheets Masters .... Vol 1 ___ Vol 2 ___ Vol 3 ___ Vol 4 ___ $9.95 _____

Structured Exercises in Wellness Promotion Series—Volumes 1-4

___ Wellness Softcover Edition .... Vol 1 ___ Vol 2 ___ Vol 3 ___ Vol 4 ___ $29.95 _____

___ Wellness Loose-Leaf Edition .... Vol 1 ___ Vol 2 ___ Vol 3 ___ Vol 4 ___ $54.95 _____

___ Wellness Worksheets Masters .... Vol 1 ___ Vol 2 ___ Vol 3 ___ Vol 4 ___ $9.95 _____

Group Process Resources

___ Playful Activities for Powerful Presentations .... $19.95 _____

___ Working with Groups from Dysfunctional Families .... $19.95 _____

___ Working with Groups from Dysfunctional Families Worksheet Masters .... $ 9.95 _____

___ Working with Women's Groups .... Vol 1 ___ Vol 2 ___ $19.95 _____

___ Working with Men's Groups .... $19.95 _____

___ Wellness Activities for Youth .... Vol 1 ___ Vol 2 ___ $19.95 _____

___ Wellness Activities for Youth Worksheet Master .... Vol 1 ___ Vol 2 ___ $9.95 _____

Relaxation Audiotapes

___ BreakTime .... $ 9.95 _____

___ Countdown to Relaxation .... $ 9.95 _____

___ Daybreak/Sundown .... $ 9.95 _____

___ Daydreams 1: Getaways .... $ 9.95 _____

___ Daydreams 2: Peaceful Places .... $ 9.95 _____

___ Harmony (music only) .... $ 9.95 _____

___ Healthy Balancing .... $ 9.95 _____

___ Inner Healing .... $ 9.95 _____

___ Natural Tranquilizers .... $ 9.95 _____

___ Personal Empowering .... $ 9.95 _____

___ Relax . . . Let Go . . . Relax .... $ 9.95 _____

___ Serenity (music only) .... $ 9.95 _____

___ Spiritual Centering .... $ 9.95 _____

___ StressRelease .... $ 9.95 _____

___ Take a Deep Breath .... $ 9.95 _____

___ Tranquility (music only) .... $ 9.95 _____

___ Warm and Heavy .... $ 9.95 _____

___ Wilderness DD 1: Canoe/Rain .... $ 9.95 _____

___ Wilderness DD 2: Island/Spring .... $ 9.95 _____

___ Wilderness DD 3: Campfire/Stream .... $ 9.95 _____

___ Wilderness DD 4: Sailboat/Pond .... $ 9.95 _____

Relaxation Resources

___ 30 Scripts—Volume 1 .... $19.95 _____

___ 30 Scripts—Volume 2 .... $19.95 _____

___ Inquire Within .... $19.95 _____

My check is enclosed. **(US funds only)**

Please charge my_____Visa _____Mastercard

#_____

Exp date _____

Signature _____

SUBTOTAL _____

TAX (MN residents 6.5%) _____

7% GST-Canadian customers only _____

**SHIPPING _____

GRAND TOTAL _____

800-247-6789

** **SHIPPING.** $5.00 ($8.00 outside U.S.)
Please call us for quotes on UPS 3rd Day,
2nd Day or Next Day Air.

ORDER FORM

Name _____

Address _____

City _____

State/Zip _____

Area Code/Telephone _____

Please make checks payable to:
Whole Person Associates Inc
210 West Michigan
Duluth MN 55802-1908
FAX: 1-218-727-0505
TOLL FREE: 1-800-247-6789

Books / Workshops-In-A-Book
____ Kicking Your Stress Habits .... $14.95 _____
____ Seeking Your Healthy Balance .... $14.95 _____

Structured Exercises in Stress Management Series—Volumes 1-4
____ Stress Softcover Edition .... Vol 1 ___ Vol 2 ___ Vol 3 ___ Vol 4 ___ $29.95 _____
____ Stress Loose-Leaf Edition .... Vol 1 ___ Vol 2 ___ Vol 3 ___ Vol 4 ___ $54.95 _____
____ Stress Worksheets Masters .... Vol 1 ___ Vol 2 ___ Vol 3 ___ Vol 4 ___ $9.95 _____

Structured Exercises in Wellness Promotion Series—Volumes 1-4
____ Wellness Softcover Edition .... Vol 1 ___ Vol 2 ___ Vol 3 ___ Vol 4 ___ $29.95 _____
____ Wellness Loose-Leaf Edition .... Vol 1 ___ Vol 2 ___ Vol 3 ___ Vol 4 ___ $54.95 _____
____ Wellness Worksheets Masters .... Vol 1 ___ Vol 2 ___ Vol 3 ___ Vol 4 ___ $9.95 _____

Group Process Resources
____ Playful Activities for Powerful Presentations .... $19.95 _____
____ Working with Groups from Dysfunctional Families .... $19.95 _____
____ Working with Groups from Dysfunctional Families Worksheet Masters .... $ 9.95 _____
____ Working with Women's Groups .... Vol 1 ___ Vol 2 ___ $19.95 _____
____ Working with Men's Groups .... $19.95 _____
____ Wellness Activities for Youth .... Vol 1 ___ Vol 2 ___ $19.95 _____
____ Wellness Activities for Youth Worksheet Master .... Vol 1 ___ Vol 2 ___ $9.95 _____

Relaxation Audiotapes
____ BreakTime .... $ 9.95 _____
____ Countdown to Relaxation .... $ 9.95 _____
____ Daybreak/Sundown .... $ 9.95 _____
____ Daydreams 1: Getaways .... $ 9.95 _____
____ Daydreams 2: Peaceful Places .... $ 9.95 _____
____ Harmony (music only) .... $ 9.95 _____
____ Healthy Balancing .... $ 9.95 _____
____ Inner Healing .... $ 9.95 _____
____ Natural Tranquilizers .... $ 9.95 _____
____ Personal Empowering .... $ 9.95 _____
____ Relax . . . Let Go . . . Relax .... $ 9.95 _____
____ Serenity (music only) .... $ 9.95 _____
____ Spiritual Centering .... $ 9.95 _____
____ StressRelease .... $ 9.95 _____
____ Take a Deep Breath .... $ 9.95 _____
____ Tranquility (music only) .... $ 9.95 _____
____ Warm and Heavy .... $ 9.95 _____
____ Wilderness DD 1: Canoe/Rain .... $ 9.95 _____
____ Wilderness DD 2: Island/Spring .... $ 9.95 _____
____ Wilderness DD 3: Campfire/Stream .... $ 9.95 _____
____ Wilderness DD 4: Sailboat/Pond .... $ 9.95 _____

Relaxation Resources
____ 30 Scripts—Volume 1 .... $19.95 _____
____ 30 Scripts—Volume 2 .... $19.95 _____
____ Inquire Within .... $19.95 _____

My check is enclosed. **(US funds only)**

Please charge my_____Visa _____Mastercard

_____

Exp date _____

Signature _____

SUBTOTAL _____
TAX (MN residents 6.5%) _____
7% GST-Canadian customers only _____
***SHIPPING** _____
GRAND TOTAL _____

800-247-6789

** **SHIPPING**. $5.00 ($8.00 outside U.S.)
Please call us for quotes on UPS 3rd Day,
2nd Day or Next Day Air.

About Whole Person Associates

At Whole Person Associates, we're 100% committed to providing stress and wellness materials that involve participants and have a "whole person" focus—body, mind, spirit, and relationships.

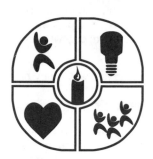

That's our mission and it's very important to us—but it doesn't tell the whole story. Behind the products in our catalog is a company full of people—and *that's* what really makes us who we are.

ABOUT THE OWNERS

Whole Person Associates was created by the vision of two people: Donald A. Tubesing, PhD, and Nancy Loving Tubesing, EdD. Since way back in 1970, Don and Nancy have been active in the stress management / wellness movement—consulting, leading seminars, writing, and publishing. Most of our early products were the result of their creativity and expertise.

Living proof that you can "stay evergreen," Don and Nancy remain the driving force behind the company and are still very active in developing new products that touch people's lives.

ABOUT THE COMPANY

Whole Person Associates was "born" in Duluth, Minnesota, and we remain committed to our lovely city on the shore of Lake Superior. All of our operations are here, which makes communication between departments much easier!

We've grown since our beginnings, but at a steady pace—we're interested in sustainable growth that allows us to keep our down-to-earth orientation—and put the same high quality into every product we offer.

ABOUT OUR EMPLOYEES

Speaking of down-to-earth, that's a requirement for each and every one of our employees. We're all product consultants, which means that anyone who answers the phone can probably answer your questions (if they can't, they'll find someone who can.)

We focus on helping you find the products that fit your needs. And we've found that the best way to do that is to hire friendly and resourceful people.

©1994 Whole Person Press 210 W Michigan Duluth MN 55802   (800) 247-6789

ABOUT OUR ASSOCIATES

Who are the "associates" in Whole Person Associates? They're the trainers, authors, musicians, and others who have developed much of the material you see on these pages. We're always on the lookout for high-quality products that reflect our "whole person" philosophy and fill a need for our customers.

Most of our products were developed by experts who are the tops in their fields, and we're very proud to be associated with them.

ABOUT OUR CUSTOMERS

Finally, we wouldn't have a reason to exist without you, our customers. We've met some of you, and we've talked to many more of you on the phone. We are always aware that without you, there would be no Whole Person Associates.

That's why we'd love to hear from you! Let us know what you think of our products—how you use them in your work, what additional products you'd like to see, and what shortcomings you've noted. Write us or call on our toll-free line. We're waiting for your call!